Dyslexia: An Introductory Guide

Dyslexia:
An Introductory
Guide

J Doyle

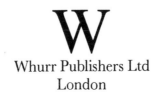

Whurr Publishers Ltd
London

© 1996 Whurr Publishers Ltd
First published 1996 by
Whurr Publishers Ltd
19b Compton Terrace, London N1 2UN, England

British Library Cataloguing in Publication Data
A catalogue record for this book is available from the British Library.

ISBN 1-897635-67-2

Printed and bound in the UK by Athenaeum Press Ltd, Gateshead, Tyne & Wear

Contents

Acknowledgements

Thanks are due to:–

- Dr Kathleen Henry (former Course Tutor at the University of Manchester) for inspiring my initial interest in dyslexia.
- Ms Julia Evans (formerly a teacher at an LEA Specific Learning Difficulties Unit) for much information and advice during eleven years of working together.
- John Wilkins (Educational Psychologist, friend and colleague) for imparting so much of his knowledge in discussions and debates.
- John Maguire (formerly a pupil at St Francis Xaviers College, Liverpool) for his assistance when the first draft of the illustrations were being prepared.
- Professor Margaret Snowling (Department of Psychology, University of York) for much valued advice and criticism of the initial text.
- The staff at Whurr Publishers for the their consideration and support.

Notes

For ease of expression throughout the book I have referred to the child as 'he' and the Teacher as 'she'. No sexism is intended by this. In each case the words 'he or she' is understood.

In early July 1995, after the main body of the text was set, the Department for Education (DFE) became the Department for Education and Employment (DFEE).

Chapter 1:
The Measurement
of Reading

A dyslexic child has difficulty with learning to read. He is also likely to have other associated difficulties such as poor spelling, slow or immature handwriting or an inability to deal with numbers, but the reading difficulty is the principal reason that makes him a cause for concern in the first place.

The question then arises as to exactly why a teacher or parent should suspect a child of being dyslexic. In fact we can leave dyslexia to one side for a moment and ask why a particular child should ever be considered to be a poor reader for any reason. In order to find an answer to any of these questions we need to know what the basic facts are regarding learning to read:

- What is a good reader?
- What is an average reader?
- Is there any means of distinguishing between them?
- If so, what is it?
- How is a poor reader identified?
- Is a dyslexic child the same as any other poor reader or is it possible that dyslexia is different in nature from other types of reading difficulty?

There *are* answers to these questions but they need to be fully explained. They can be understood only by setting the explanations into the general background which relates to such matters as the everyday teaching of reading, the differences that arise between children when they are learning to read and how the differences can be measured.

The Teaching of Reading

Each year millions of children in Britain attend school and are taught reading by hundreds of thousands of teachers. This is a practice which has applied for more than a hundred and twenty years and has proved, by and large, to be a successful one. Success can be claimed as most children leave school able to read at a level which allows them to cope quite adequately with the demands of life in present-day society.

The fact that *every* school leaver is not fully literate is very much to be regretted and is a situation which everyone involved would like to see corrected. But the positive side of the picture is quite remarkable. The fact is that most children in Britain do learn to read despite there being many differences and difficulties to be found within the child population generally and despite the fact that a number of approaches to reading are in general use. The rate of success in reading is independent of size of school and also of where the schools are located. Village schools, those in suburbs and ones in inner cities all produce literate children with more or less equal rates of success.

What happens in the case of most children is that they start to learn to read at about the age of five, having worked for some time at building up their pre-reading skills. After this they acquire more reading skills and steadily become more proficient over a period of about four years by which time, at the age of about nine, they are fully literate. By 'fully literate' we mean that they can decipher print accurately and make sense of what is written by being able to 'decode' the text of a book or newspaper. However, after the age of nine children must continue to read increasingly more difficult types of writing if they are to enlarge their vocabularies and build on the skills they have acquired. This process is illustrated in Figure 1.1.

Comparing one age-group of the child population with another, it is only to be expected that the nine-year-olds are able to read better than the eight-year-olds who, in turn, read better than seven-year-olds and so on down the age-groups. Also, the seven-year-olds of today will in a year's time be able to read as well as today's eight-year-olds. In two years from now they will be reading as competently as today's nine-year-olds and so on into the future.

It is important to be able to measure how well a child can read so that an accurate and unbiased assessment of the child's progress may be made. This is best done by using reading tests and we now need to consider these and the manner in which they are used.

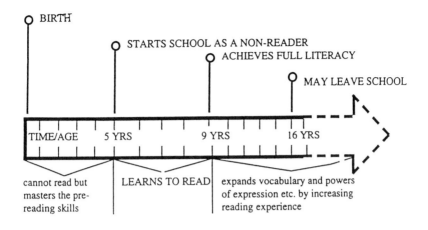

Figure 1.1: Stages in Reading Development (Ages refer to the average child)

The Measurement of Reading Progress

Over the years a large number of reading tests have been designed and developed. Comparing one with another some variety is shown. Many reading tests have been designed to be given to a whole group of children, such as a class, at the same time; others are meant to be given to an individual. Some consist of a list of single words, others consist of sentences from each of which there is a word missing which needs to be supplied or chosen from a group of possibilities.

The simplest and most straightforward reading tests are the word lists. Each of these tests consists of a number of words which need to be read in a certain order. At the start the words are short, common and easily pronounced but gradually become longer, less common and irregular. The Schonnell graded word reading test is a good example. The test starts off with words such as 'tree', 'little' and 'book' and progresses to 'ineradicable', 'fictitious' and 'idio-syncrasy'. (A few of the many reading tests that are available to teachers and others are shown in Figure 1.2). For a reading test to be of any worthwhile value it needs to be properly designed, checked and standardised otherwise the results will have little meaning. A word-list type of reading test will be brought into exist-ence by a person or a team who will start by drawing up a list of words which they assume will be suitable to determine the reading progress of children between the ages of five and fourteen. A

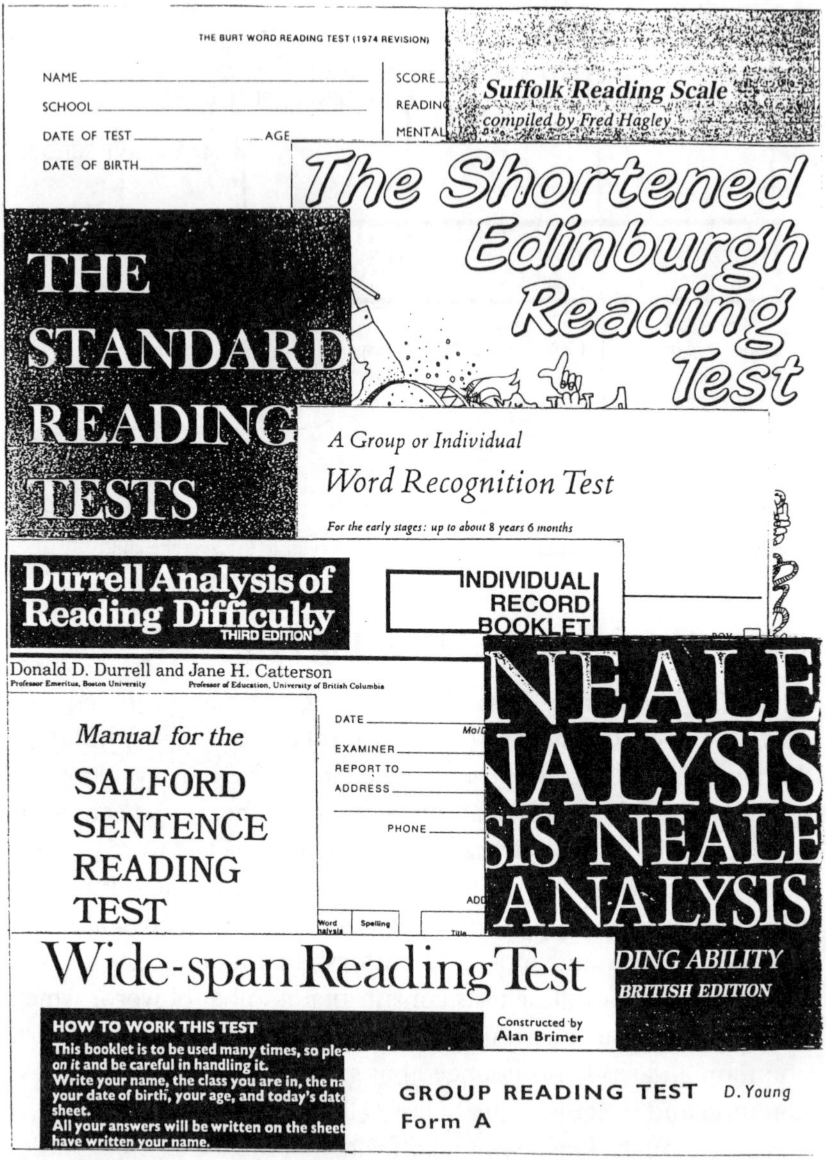

THE BURT WORD READING TEST (1974 REVISION)

NAME _____
SCHOOL _____
DATE OF TEST _____ AGE ____
DATE OF BIRTH _____

SCORE ____
READING
MENTAL

Suffolk Reading Scale
compiled by Fred Hagley

The Shortened
Edinburgh
Reading
Test

THE
STANDARD
READING
TESTS

A Group or Individual

Word Recognition Test

For the early stages: up to about 8 years 6 months

Durrell Analysis of
Reading Difficulty
THIRD EDITION

INDIVIDUAL
RECORD
BOOKLET

Donald D. Durrell and Jane H. Catterson
Professor Emeritus, Boston University   Professor of Education, University of British Columbia

Manual for the
SALFORD
SENTENCE
READING
TEST

DATE _____
EXAMINER _____
REPORT TO _____
ADDRESS _____

PHONE _____

NEALE
NALYSIS
SIS NEALE
ANALYSIS

Word Spelling
nalysis

Wide-span Reading Test

DING ABILITY
BRITISH EDITION

HOW TO WORK THIS TEST
This booklet is to be used many times, so plea
on it and be careful in handling it.
Write your name, the class you are in, the na
your date of birth, your age, and today's date
sheet.
All your answers will be written on the sheet
have written your name.

Constructed by
Alan Brimer

GROUP READING TEST   D. Young
Form A

Figure 1.2: A few of the many reading tests available

perfectly designed test would be one which is easy enough for most five-year-old children to be able to make a start on, yet still difficult enough for some fourteen-year-olds not to be able to complete. In addition it needs to be able to distinguish each of the age-groups in between; that is, children aged twelve should do better than those aged eleven who in turn will be better than the ten and nine-year-olds etc.

In other words, what needs to be avoided is the production of a reading test which is so easy that many children – even the youngest age-groups – obtain high scores, or so difficult that very few children, even the older ones, can achieve any success, or so badly designed in between the two extremes that children of different ages e.g. nine, ten and eleven, all score the same and cannot be distinguished. Needless to say, a properly designed reading test is a rather sensitive, and therefore quite accurate, measuring device and to achieve these qualities some work will need to be invested in it by the designers.

Therefore, the initial word list drawn up by the design team will need to be tested out in one or more pilot studies by using one or more groups of children. The pilot study should identify any words that are too easy, those that are too difficult and also whether any particular words have been included 'out of order', i.e. in a place either too high up or too low down on the list. A word which is found in practice to be read very easily but which has been placed between two more difficult words will need to be placed somewhere more suitable. Eventually a word list will be produced from the original which will be an improvement on what was first drawn up, as errors will have been corrected; but it will still need to be standardised. It is not sufficient simply to have a list of suitable words arranged in the correct order of difficulty and which is capable of being used on children from five to fourteen years of age. In addition to all this you still need to know how many words a given child should be expected to read. For instance, if the total list consists of 100 words, what score would you expect from an eight-year-old? From an eleven-year-old?

To obtain this information the test must be set for yet more children and this time larger numbers will need to be used than in the pilot study(ies). Ideally the test should be given to the whole population of schoolchildren but as there are so many million of them in the British Isles it would not be very easy. Therefore, groups of children are used as there is no easy alternative.

Ideally the test should be standardised on a large number of groups each containing a large number of children but in most cases this is not possible and the test design team are forced to settle for something less.

However, they do have a great deal of information about the nation's schoolchildren and they can make use of this in selecting their groups. What they will aim for is to standardise the test on a group of children who will be, as far as possible, a 'scale model' of the total population of schoolchildren. The group should have the same proportion of inner-city children, of children from ethnic minority backgrounds, of children from each of the social groups etc. as in the overall population. Provided this is done the results will be accurate to within a very small margin of error and the test can be standardised accordingly, e.g. children aged five score 5, those aged six score 12, those aged 7 score 18, etc. It cannot be emphasised too strongly just how important the process of standardisation is as part of test design. It is not much help to a teacher or parent just to know that John, aged eight, was given a reading test and was able to read 35 words correctly. What needs to be asked is whether his score is a good, average or poor achievement for a child of his age. If most other children of John's age can score only 20 then he is doing well – but if they are scoring 50 the picture is a very different one.

The Schonnell Test mentioned above was revised in 1971 by being standardised on 10 000 children in Salford. It was found that the average seven-year-old read 15 words, eight-year-olds read 30 words, and so on. (This particular test consists of 100 words and is capable of measuring the reading ages of children from below six to above twelve years).

The Pattern of Children's Reading Scores

We now need to examine the picture that is produced when a properly designed and well-standardised reading test is used on large numbers of children. Imagine that there is such a test, which we will call the 'Smith and Jones' Reading Test and the Department for Education (DFE) decides to use it in order to assess the reading ability of the country's seven-year-olds. There could be many good reasons for carrying out such a survey. The DFE might want to see how well today's seven-year-olds compare with those of last year, or five years or even ten years ago. It might want the information to use as a basis for comparing future seven-year-olds in time to come.

Whatever the reason, the survey should ideally include all seven-year-olds but considering that there would be more than 700 000 of them it will probably be considered that this number would be too large to organise and that only a proportion should be used. It could be agreed that 100 000 would be sufficient to provide the information required and so this number is settled on. Other arrangements would then follow. Out of all 700 000 children due to reach the age of seven during the year planned for the survey it could be arranged for the 100 000 required to be chosen completely at random by means of a computer and for each child to be tested in school on their birthday or within a week either side of it. At the end of the year there would then be information available on 100 000 children who represented one-seventh or so of the country's seven-year-olds and who should be exactly like the total population of 700 000 in every other respect. There should be the same proportions of girls to boys, of city dwellers to those from rural areas, of children from ethnic minority backgrounds, etc.

The result obtained from each child would be a number representing how many words from the 'Smith and Jones' Reading Test the child was able to read. Obviously, 100 000 results is a large amount of information to cope with and make sense of. Decisions would need to be made as to how to get it all down on paper.

Listing the Results

The simplest way would be to draw up a list of the names of the 100 000 children and put next to each name the number of words correctly read by that child, but this would result in a large number of sheets of paper, probably bound into a booklet of about 1000 pages it if were possible to put details of 100 children on each page.

Tabling the Results

A better way would be to ignore the details of individual children and instead to count them in groups. For instance, a count could be made of the number of children who were not able to read any words, how many could read just one word, how many two, and so on down the list until the greatest number of words read was reached. (In our example this is 30). After all, it is not necessary to know the names of the children involved so the listing of each child individually as in the first method would result in a large quantity of totally irrelevant information by which no purpose is served. Counting the number of children able to read each given number of words would summarise all of the important details very neatly into one sheet of paper and information could be gained at a glance.

This has been done in Table 1.1. Essentially there are five columns of figures. In the first column is a list of the number of words read and this runs from 0 to 30. The second column sets out how many children could read each given number of words. The third column tells us the same as column 2 but gives the children as a percentage of the total. Columns 4 and 5 are very useful as they tell you how many children can read any given number of words or less. (Column 4 gives the information as a number and

Table 1.1: 'Smith and Jones' Reading Test: results obtained from children aged 7.0 years (total children – 100 000)

1 Words read	2 Children	3 (% of total)	4 Cumulative total of children	5 Cumulative % of children
0	129	0.1	129	0.1
1	151	0.2	280	0.3
2	242	0.2	522	0.5
3	402	0.4	924	0.9
4	634	0.6	1558	1.5
5	964	1.0	2522	2.5
6	1419	1.4	3941	3.9
7	2018	2.0	5959	6.0
8	2760	2.7	8719	8.7
9	3702	3.7	12421	12.4
10	4672	4.7	17093	17.1
11	5688	5.7	22781	22.8
12	6824	6.8	29605	29.6
13	7734	7.7	37339	37.3
14	8330	8.3	45669	45.7
15	8662	8.7	54331	54.3
16	8321	8.3	62653	62.7

the table continues

| 30 | 88 | 0.1 | 100000 | 100 |

column 5 gives it as a percentage). Looking at the table we see from the top line that only 129 children out of the total were not able to read any words at all (0) and this comparatively small number was only one-tenth of 1% of the population (0.1%).

We see for instance that 5 words were read by 964 children (or 1%) of the total. However the number of children who could read *5 or less* words was 2522 (2.5%). The figure of 2522 was obtained by adding those who read 0 words (129) to those who read 1 (151) to those who read 2 (242), 3 (402), 4 (634) and 5 (964). Hence 129+151+242+ 402+634+964 = 2522 (2.5%). The number 2522 is the *cumulative total* of children reading 5 words or less.

The most important point to be appreciated from the results of this imaginary survey is that despite the fact that all the children were of the same age they did not all produce the same results! In fact a very wide range of results is seen, with a few children not able to read at all yet some others able to proceed right through to as many as 30 words.

However, the most important thing that this survey tells us is that for seven-year-olds the ability to read *15* words on this particular reading list has significance. Why this is so can be understood from Column 5. As can be seen, 14 words or less can be read by about 46% of the population and this is less than half. By the same token *more than half* of the population (54%) can read 15 words or more and so the 'expected' or 'normal' score for a seven-year-old on this reading test is 15. At any stage in a child's education it is to be expected that a child will perform at the same level as most other children of the same age and so a score of 15 or more will be expected from any seven-year-old who is given this test. We should add that this is what will be expected *provided that all other things in the child's life are equal.* Often they are not equal, however, but we will be considering that matter at a later stage.

Graphing the Results

A third way of presenting the results so that they may be accurately analysed would be to take Columns 1 and 2 from the table and draw a graph from them. Along the bottom of the graph would be set out the contents of Column 1, the number of words read and which would need to run from 0 to 30. Up the side of the graph would be Column 2, the number of children at each number of words and this would best run from 0 to 9000 in order to accommodate the actual range of 129 – 8662.

The graph would appear as in Figure 1.3(a). If we scan across the graph from left to right we see that it is curved with a high point in the middle and falls away in a regular manner on either side, one half of the graph being a 'mirror image' of the other.

The score of 15 is all-important because:

- the peak of the graph is directly above it, showing that 15 is the most 'popular' score as more children obtain that exact score than any other;
- more than half of all the children tested scored 15 or above;
- most children are grouped around the score of 15 and so are in a fairly close range of it. There are many fewer at the extreme ends of the graph in the 'low score' and 'high score' ranges.

Because a score of 15 on our 'Smith and Jones' Reading Test has proved to be so very significant in the case of seven-year-old children it is perfectly in order for teachers, parents and others to regard this score as A READING AGE OF EXACTLY 7 YRS 0 MTHS and this is what is done in order to make results more meaningful. To say that seven-year-old John has had his reading ability tested and he scored 15 tells us very little. To say that he proved to have a reading age of 7;0 tells us a great deal as a *compar-*

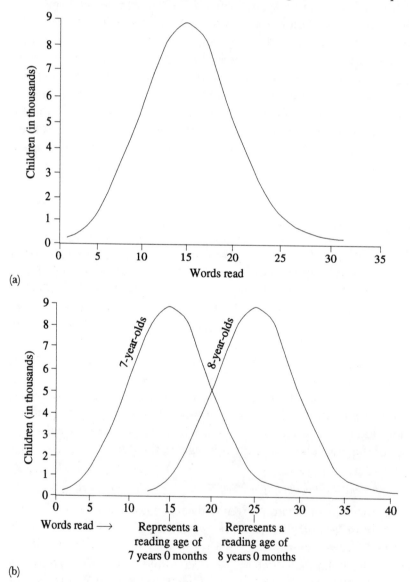

(a)

(b)

Figure 1.3 (a) Graph of results obtained from giving reading test to 100,000 seven-year-olds, and (b) Graphs comparing reading abilities of 7- and 8-year-olds

ison can now be made between John himself and other children in the country of the same age. It is only with *this* information (a reading age) that we are able to judge how well or badly he can read.

Testing Other Age-groups

So far in our imaginary reading survey we have concentrated on a single age-group: seven-year-olds. But much can be learned by testing other age-groups and making a comparison. If the same procedure that was carried out on seven-year-olds was also applied to the country's eight-year-olds, and the graph which resulted was to be drawn on the same framework (axes) as that of the seven-year-olds then the result would be as in Figure 1.3(b).

The graph relating to the eight-year-olds is seen to be identical to that of the seven-year-olds but lies to the right of it, the 'peak' for the older children being at the 25-word level which is 10 greater than that for the younger ones.

This should not be a surprise. The eight-year-olds, having had an extra year at school, will naturally be able to read more than the seven-year-olds. Just as a score of 15 represents a reading age of 7;0 years, in the same way a score of 25 represents a reading age of 8;0 years. Furthermore, the two groups of children are found to 'overlap' to a certain extent, the more able of the younger children being as competent at reading as are the less able of the older ones. The two age-groups of children are not completely separate in their reading abilities, there being some of each group at the same levels of competence.

It is easy to appreciate that if the process were to be continued with older groups of children and graphs were to be drawn relating also to nine-, ten- and eleven-year-old children then a *series* of graphs would result, each successive one lying to the right of that of the age-groups immediately below it but at the same time *overlapping* those on either side. In the same way, the particular number of words read, which was marked by the peak of each age-group's graph, could be easily identified and 'converted' into the particular reading age. The result would be as set out in Figure 1.4.

When the graphs produced by a sufficient number of different age-groups are assembled together in this manner it is possible to view the bottom line of the graph as a ladder lying on its side and with the rungs numbered in order from the foot (which lies to the left) to the top (at the right). Particular rungs are then marked to represent reading ages, e.g. rung 15 being reading age 7;0, as in our

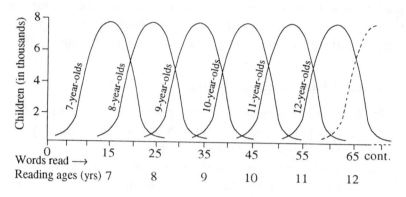

Figure 1.4 Graphs comparing reading abilities of consecutive age-groups

'Smith and Jones' Reading Test. When the ladder is set upright a child undergoing a reading test can be thought of as starting to 'climb' the ladder and it can then be seen just how 'high' he is able to climb. Each marked rung would show the height which *most* children of that age-group are able to reach. Most nine-year-olds will reach the 9 years rung (number 35 in our example) but some will not be able to achieve this just as some others will be able to 'climb' even higher. The rungs of the imaginary ladder will act as reading ages for the children involved. This is shown in Figure 1.5.

Summary

We began this chapter by saying that as dyslexia involved difficulties with reading it was necessary for all concerned with the problem to have a clear idea in their minds as to how a dyslexic child could be identified from others.

A number of questions were asked and we are now in a position to answer many of them. The questions were:

- *What is a good reader?* We now know that any child who is considered to be a good reader is able to read *better* than most children of the same age as himself. This can be proved by the child obtaining a 'high' mark on reading test which in turn shows that he has a 'high' reading age.
- *What is an average reader?* One who is capable of reading at the *same* level as most children of his age.
- *Is there any means of distinguishing between them? If so, what is it?* By giving each a reading test which has been properly designed and accurately standardised on samples of the particular population of children for which it was intended.

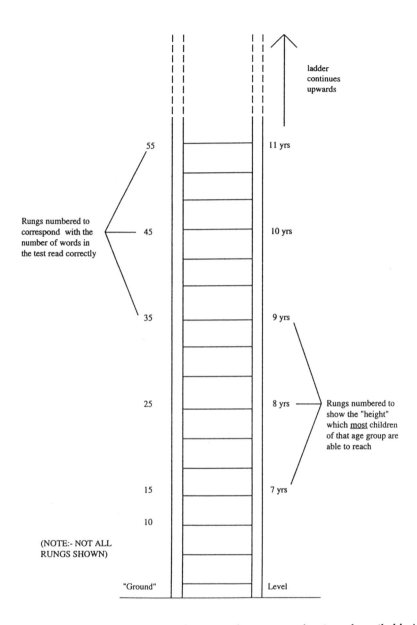

Figure 1.5 Diagram to illustrate how a reading test may be viewed as a 'ladder' a child can 'climb'

- *How is a poor reader identified?* From the score obtained on a reading test of the type described.

  (Before we proceed to the last question it will be appreciated that the important task of identifying children with reading difficulties is something which can be undertaken in an efficient and unbiased manner using an appropriate reading test.

Teachers, parents and others do *not* need to rely on their own impressions, hunches or suspicions in the matter as these can often be quite misleading. Any worries about a child's reading abilities should be settled at the earliest opportunity by the use of a test).

* *Is a dyslexic child the same as any other poor reader or is it possible that dyslexia is different in nature from other types of reading difficulties?* Nothing we have covered so far can provide an answer to this question. The information we will require in order to give us the answer will be dealt with in the coming chapters.

Now that we know something about how reading progress is measured we go on in the following chapter to discuss what influences can affect a child's reading progress, the different difficulties that can arise and the manner in which they operate.

Chapter 2:
Reading Difficulties
Explained

The single most important piece of information which the previous chapter dealt with is that NOT ALL SCHOOL-AGE CHILDREN HAVE THE SAME READING ABILITY but show quite wide variation. Although most children are within average range nevertheless there is a certain percentage (say 15–20%) who are below average, and a similar amount above.

This situation is, of course, quite common knowledge and hardly needs to be stated but it does not answer the burning question as to WHY this should be so. Just why can't all children show the same progress in reading? What are the reasons for it? Can we detect them? Can anything be done to help matters? These questions are very important to us in our attempts to reach an understanding of dyslexia. If a situation such as this exists there must be reasons for it and we need to do our best to uncover them. If a group of children – a school full, say – do not all have the same level of competence in reading then logically there can be only one explanation:- THERE ARE INFLUENCES INVOLVED WHICH PRODUCE CHANGE. These influences must be

either (a) causing the reading ability of some children to become *better* than that of others;

or (b) causing it to become *worse* in some than in others;

or (c) acting to cause *both* effects.

We now need to examine everything we know that is part of a child's present make-up, history or social background and which could possibly affect his reading ability in one direction or the other. Before we go on to that topic it might be helpful to mention some factors that need not necessarily affect reading ability so that they may be cleared out of the way and prevent possible future confusion.

Location of School

Neither the general nor the particular location of a school should prevent children from learning to read adequately. Children in all parts of Britain are found to master the skill. England, Scotland, Wales and the Isle of Man all produce literate children. Schools are located in a wide variety of geographical settings: in highland communities, on small islands, as part of pit villages, big cities and towns. However, although full literacy can be achieved by a child in any of these settings there are some differences between one and the other with respect to *average* results.

Social Class

The ability of a child to read does not depend directly on the occupation of the parents or the level of income which the family have. It is possible for good. average and poor readers to be found in all social groupings. However, *general* differences are to be found, with children from higher social groupings tending to produce better results than others.

Gender

Boys and girls are both capable of achieving full literacy, but differences are displayed in the process. Generally speaking, girls tend to learn to read at a faster rate than do boys so that within any particular year group the reading ability of the girls will be found to be somewhat better, on average, than that of the boys.

None of these three factors has a profound influence on the ability to read, any more than does height, weight, eye colour or blood group. There are other aspects of children's development also mistakeny considered by some to cause difficulties with reading but the three above are the ones most commonly placed in this category.

Factors which Influence Reading

And now to examine those factors which definitely *do* have a part to play in the way a child's reading skills develop. In Figure 2.1 there is a list of 20 causes (or factors) which have been set down in alphabetical order. This list contains all the influences most commonly considered by people working in education to play a part. (However, no claim is being made that the list is exhaustive; over time other influences could well be discovered).

By way of explanation it should be said that when primary school teachers attend courses relating to the teaching of reading they are often asked to produce their own lists of what they consider causes reading difficulties. The list produced here is the result of putting a number of these lists together, so we can be reassured that we are not dealing with unreal, high-flown theory but rather down-to-earth basic facts. Real teachers who are working every day in the nation's schools are able, from long experience, to identify what applies and what does not. Their opinions are confirmed by others working with children in the education system. Our list can be analysed in a number of different ways, each of which provides us with useful information. It would be useful for us to know, for instance:

- What influence each has on a child's reading progress: positive, neutral or negative?
- Whether a particular factor influences all children or only some.
- Where the difficulties are to be found: within the child? Within the home background? Within the school?
- Which agencies should be consulted? And which can provide support?
- How quickly can any particular difficulty be detected after onset?
- How serious an effect is there likely to be on the child's reading ability: short term/medium term/long term?

We shall consider the first of these classifications as, at this stage at least, it is the most informative. We need to be clear that as a first step in getting to understand children's reading difficulties we are considering *any influence at all* that has a bearing on children's reading progress, and so are just as interested in anything capable of improving reading ability as we are in anything that does the opposite. Once we have become acquainted with the contents of the whole field we can look more closely at those factors which cause reading progress to be held back.

Types of Influence

When we do analyse the list into the types of influence on children's reading we find that there are three distinct categories, those being:

1.   AGE;
2.   INTELLIGENCE;
3.   The other 18.

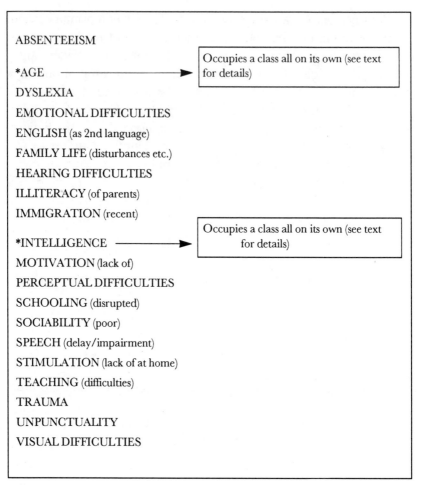

ABSENTEEISM

*AGE ——————————————▶ Occupies a class all on its own (see text for details)

DYSLEXIA

EMOTIONAL DIFFICULTIES

ENGLISH (as 2nd language)

FAMILY LIFE (disturbances etc.)

HEARING DIFFICULTIES

ILLITERACY (of parents)

IMMIGRATION (recent)

*INTELLIGENCE ——————————▶ Occupies a class all on its own (see text for details)

MOTIVATION (lack of)

PERCEPTUAL DIFFICULTIES

SCHOOLING (disrupted)

SOCIABILITY (poor)

SPEECH (delay/impairment)

STIMULATION (lack of at home)

TEACHING (difficulties)

TRAUMA

UNPUNCTUALITY

VISUAL DIFFICULTIES

Figure 2.1 Factors which can affect reading progress in children

AGE occupies a class all on its own. It relates positively to reading progress as an increase in age leads to an increase in reading ability, ten-year-olds being able to read better than nine-year-olds who, in turn, read better than eight-year-olds etc. Age is unique as it is the only one of the 20 factors listed which:

(a)   affects every child *and*
(b)   does so to the same degree, year on year.

When comparing one child with another it is to be expected that an older child will be able to read better than a younger child. Many comparisons of one child with another can be made in a meaningful way only if the children are of the same age, thereby removing the age factor. (More will be said of this later).

INTELLIGENCE also occupies a class on its own, being different from age and also different from the other 18 factors. Intelligence is unique because it is the only one of the 20 which:

(a)   affects all children *and*
(b)   is capable of relating to reading ability in three different ways. Intelligence can relate *positively* (in being above average and contributing to a high reading age), or in a *neutral* way (by being of average range and so producing an average reading age) or *negatively* (by being below average and causing the child's reading age to be low).

THE OTHER 18 can all be grouped together into one category as they all have two characteristics in common:

(a)   Each relates in a *negative* manner to a child's reading ability, causing it to be lower than it would otherwise be.
(b)   Each factor affects only a small proportion of the total population of children.

The results are summarised in Table 2.1. The contents of this table serve to give us the information we require about factors which influence reading ability and which we mentioned at the start of the chapter. We can see from the table that all three possible types of influence are at work. There is one causing the reading ability of some to be *better* than others (age), a number causing it to be *worse* (the group of 18) and one that is capable of acting both ways (intelligence).

Table 2.1				
		Type of influence (summary)		
		Positive	Neutral	Negative
	All	Age	–	–
Proportion of children affected		- - - - - - - - Intelligence		- - - - - - - -
		High	Average	Low
	Some	–	–	Absenteeism etc.. ↓ Visual Difficulties (18 in total)

Analysing the Problems of Poor Reading

So far in this chapter we have learned that:

- there are at least 20 factors at work in a child's make-up, history or social background which can influence his reading ability;
- these 20 fall into three distinct groupings, and that
- the twenty, between them, can act in three different ways on the child's reading.

All this makes for a rather complex picture and so when we come to consider an individual child we need to pick our way very carefully through the details of the case as we know them in order to arrive at an accurate analysis of his difficulties. In the first place it is easy to make the mistake of not giving proper allowance for age. It is quite common for parents to be worried about the reading progress of their seven-year-old child because he is not reading as well as his nine-year-old sister. This demonstrates a *real difference* in reading ability between two children but does not automatically mean that there is any kind of *difficulty*. It is quite possible that each child is reading at an average level for the individual's age-group and that neither child is experiencing any difficulty. It is reasonable to suppose that when the younger brother attains the present age of his older sister he will be able then to read as well as she is doing now. A difference is *not* a difficulty if it can be accounted for by AGE.

But of course even within a group of children all of the same age there are poor readers and when these are considered they are found to fall into two groups:

1.   Those whose reading level is capable of being higher than it is at present but is prevented from being so by a particular difficulty (or combination of difficulties). (The difficulty(ies) will be found in the group of 18 in the bottom left-hand box of Table 2.1. Each of these affect only a small proportion of children but always retard, or hold back, their reading progress).
2.   Those children who do not have any particular difficulty(ies) but are still not able to read as well as most other children of their own age. Although they do not have a particular difficulty these children do show a *difference* between themselves and others in their age bracket.

These two groups of poor readers are the product of two different types of influence or force which act on the general population of schoolchildren. This is only to be expected. Having removed AGE from the analysis at the beginning of the process by considering and comparing only children of the same age we are left with INTELLI-GENCE and THE GROUP OF 18. The effects of the latter produce the group of children with reading ages lower than they ought to be, and the effects of intelligence (low, in these cases) produce the children who are at the bottom end of the scale.

The child with the reading difficulty caused by one of the 18 factors is understood to be capable of achieving better, and better progress will be made in reading once the difficulty involved is detected and cured/corrected/remediated/improved/prevented. There is the concept that a child has a certain level of potential which the particular factor is presently preventing the child from reaching (visual difficulties, hearing impairment and absenteeism are good examples).

The child who displays no difficulties whatsoever but still achieves below average is considered to have a lower level of potential than the others but to be reading to the limit it allows. This type of child is usually found to be performing at a similar low level in most other areas of school work, therefore confirming the overall picture.

Where Difficulties Arise

When the 20 factors known to influence a child's reading progress are grouped according to where they originate it is seen that there are only three sources, the child himself, the home background and the school. The child accounts for 10 of them, the home for another nine and the school for just one. Table 2.2 shows which factor can be grouped under which heading. We will now mention each one briefly with the exceptions of age, intelligence and dyslexia. The first two we have discussed earlier and dyslexia has a whole chapter devoted to it later.

Table 2.2: Where reading influences originate		
Within child	Within family	Within school
Age	Absenteeism	Teaching (difficulties)
Dyslexia	English (2nd language)	
Emotional difficulties	Family life (disturbed)	
Hearing	Illiteracy (of parents)	
Intelligence	Immigration (recent)	
Motivation	Schooling (disrupted)	
Perception	Stimulation (poor at home)	
Sociability	Trauma	
Speech	Unpunctuality	
Vision		

Absenteeism: No child will make progress in reading unless he is in school available be taught. Generally speaking, the greater the absenteeism the less will be the progress made.

Emotional difficulties: The extremely sensitive or very insecure child will be such that his emotional state acts as a barrier to learning. Sensitive handling will be required on the part of the school and in extreme cases outside opinion may need to be consulted.

English as a second language: When this is the situation in a family a child who is learning to read is likely to be at a disadvantage. In many families the background knowledge of English which the other children in the class have will be lacking. Reading could take longer to get established.

Family life disturbances: Unfortunately some children are in families that do not have a settled existence. Frequent changes of address during the early years of schooling, particularly when the child has to change schools as a result, can cause underachievement. Even when a change of school does not feature, disturbances which lead to the child often having a broken night's sleep or needing to spend time away from home with relatives can contribute to a child's reading progress being less than it should.

Hearing: A child may have imperfect hearing in one or both ears and the degree of hearing difficulty can show wide variation. Any hearing difficulty will produce difficulties at school, particularly in relation to reading. Much can be done to remedy hearing difficulties which makes early detection vital.

Illiteracy of parents: Any young school-age child is placed at a big disadvantage if his parents cannot read. Much encouragement in reading comes from the home. The child who cannot have stories read to him by his parents, or be listened to when he is reading out loud, is bound to be hindered in his attempts to progress.

Immigration (recent): The young child who has recently arrived in the UK from a different culture – particularly one where a different language is spoken – will need some time to adapt to the new culture in general and school life in particular.

Motivation: Most children are keen to read but a small proportion lack this drive. This could be for a number of reasons, often quite complex, and will normally need investigation if attempts by the school to encourage the child do not succeed.

Perception: In certain cases a child can have adequate eyesight and hearing and yet not always be able to make proper sense of what he is looking at or listening to. For example, a letter of the alphabet can be interpreted by the child as facing the opposite way to what it actually is. Perceptional difficulties can lead to reading difficulties and justify further investigation.

Schooling (disrupted): In an ideal world each child would attend just one primary school where he would be happy and would achieve. Happily most children are in this category but a proportion have the continuity of their primary education disrupted by needing to change schools, sometimes more than once. This can have an adverse effect on a child's progress as he settles into a different school and classroom routine as well as adapting to a different teacher.

Sociability: Some children display a poor ability to socialise with others and settle into the school routine. At one extreme are withdrawn, shy, under-reactive children and at the other boisterous, outgoing, aggressive types. All children need a settling-in period but if a particular child shows difficulties for a prolonged period then additional support is likely to be required.

Speech: Any difficulties with speech will affect a child's reading progress. Speech may be delayed, immature or have some kind of defect such as a stammer or stutter. In reading, any child not able to pronounce a word properly will be disadvantaged and is likely to experience a delay in the development of his reading skills. In moderate or severe cases a speech therapist's opinion should be sought.

Stimulation (poor at home): Unfortunately some children are from homes where there is little intellectual stimulation for them. Conversation is lacking, books, stimulating toys and other materials are in short supply or non-existent. Any child from such a home will undoubtedly find it more difficult to cope with reading and other school work as a smooth start often depends on the child's experiences and variety of stimulation in the pre-school years.

Teaching (difficulties): On occasions a class in a primary school can be unfortunate enough to experience a change of teacher part way through the school year. Sometimes, if the regular class teacher is absent on a long-term basis, the class can be taught by a succession of supply teachers, depending on the exact circumstances under which the school is operating. Such a state of affairs is to be avoided if at all possible as the progress of children is quite likely to suffer as a result.

Trauma: If a child suffers an accident or experiences the death of a close relative, there can be a period of time afterwards, often quite lengthy, in which school progress will suffer. All possible allowances will need to be made for such a child but any ground lost should eventually be made up.

Unpunctuality: Any child regularly late for school, even though putting in a full attendance, is likely to be missing out on opportunities to develop his reading skills. Action should be taken in all cases by the education welfare officer for the school and support might need to be given to certain families so as to encourage regular attendance by the child.

Vision: Some children have difficulties related to vision but fortunately most of these are not serious and can easily be corrected once detected. There could be longsightedness, shortsightedness, astigmatism, lack of acuity in one or both eyes or a squint (strabismus) in one or both eyes. Early detection is important as good vision is essential for reading progress.

Support Agencies

Fortunately we have a society where there are numerous agencies available to assist children with any of a variety of difficulties. Sometimes these agencies may be undermanned, under-resourced and overworked but at least they exist and may be called on to assist the child with reading difficulties. Table 2.3 shows the particular professional personnel that can be called on to advise and support in the case of each of the difficulties we have described in this chapter. The three main agencies involved are the Local Education Authority (LEA), the Area Health Authority (AHA) and Social Services (SS) but others also contribute. The range of services available will vary from one part of the country to another and the exact title used will, in some cases, be different from those used here but most if not all should be available wherever a child in difficulties might live. Although it is possible to analyse the difficulties in other ways, those which we have covered here are primarily the most productive and informative. It would be useful to know also such things as the degree to which a child can be affected in each case, how readily each type can be detected etc., but questions such as these are, by their nature, difficult to answer with any high degree of accuracy so no further analyses will be attempted here. Another complicating factor is that it is possible for a child to experience a number of difficulties at the same time, so in those cases the effects are likely to be more marked and the remedies more difficult to put into practice.

Summary

To summarise the chapter:

- A child's progress in reading is affected by two universal influences: age and intelligence. These are so described because they affect *all* children. Progress may also be affected by one or more other influences related to *either* the child, *or* the home/social background, *or* the school. These affect only some children. Dyslexia is one of these other influences and is dealt with fully in this book.

- Intelligence is a very significant influence on reading because it can contribute a great deal to a child being able to read *better* than most others of his age, as well as having the opposite effect.

- We need to be aware of the difference between a child not reading as well as others in his age-group due to the influence of intelligence, and a child not being able to read as well as he should due to other reasons, such as those shown in the Table 2.3.

Table 2.3 showing supportive professionals and their employing bodies										
	L.E.A					A.H.A		S.S	OTHER	
	EP	EWO	SpT	PSP	Sch	CMO	SpTh	SoWk	CG	LC
Absenteeism	–	●	–	–	–	–	–	–	–	–
Emotional difficulties	●	–	–	–	–	–	–	–	–	–
English (2nd lang)	–	–	●	●	–	–	–	–	●	●
Family Life (disrupted)	–	–	–	●	–	–	–	●	–	–
Hearing	–	–	–	–	–	●	–	–	–	–
Illiteracy (of parents)	–	–	–	●	–	–	–	–	●	●
Immigration (recent)	–	–	–	–	–	–	–	●	●	–
Motivation	●	–	–	–	–	–	–	–	–	–
Perception	●	●	–	–	–	–	–	–	–	–
Schooling (disrupted)	–	●	–	●	–	–	–	●	–	–
Sociability	●	–	–	–	–	–	–	–	–	–
Speech (difficulties)	●	–	–	–	–	–	●	–	–	–
Stimulation (poor at home)	–	–	–	●	●	–	–	●	–	–
Teaching (difficulties)	–	–	–	–	●	–	–	–	–	–
Trauma	●	–	–	●	–	–	–	●	–	–
Unpunctuality	–	●	–	–	–	–	–	●	–	–
Vision	–	–	–	–	–	●	–	–	–	–

EP = Educational Psychologist	EWO = Educational Welfare Officer
SpT = Specialist Teacher	PSP = Parental Support Project
Sch = School	CMO = Clinical Medical Officer
SpTh = Speech Therapist	SoWk = Social Worker
CG = Community Groups	LC = Local College

The former type of child is usually described as being BACKWARD at reading and the latter as being RETARDED in reading. (More will be said about this important difference in the following chapters.) Because intelligence has an influence as great as it does it needs to be explained in more detail, and this is done in the next chapter.

Chapter 3:
The Influence of
Intelligence

Intelligence plays a large part in our lives and particularly in how we learn. This applies irrespective of whether the learning we are talking about is that which takes place in an ordinary everyday manner (the means by which a great deal of our knowledge of the world and how it operates is learned) or in the formal sense, that is to say by being taught in school or trained in workshops etc.

The intelligence a child possesses will govern many aspects of the manner and ease in which new knowledge is acquired and new skills mastered. Intelligence plays a large part in the process of learning to read etc., and when attempts are made to diagnose a child's learning difficulties one of the most important and relevant pieces of information which needs to be established is just how intelligent the child is. Sensible and accurate interpretations of much of the other information acquired about the child will only be possible when carried out against a background of knowledge of the child's intelligence level.

The idea of intelligence is quite well known to us in the everyday sense of the word – it means clever, brainy, quick witted, 'fast on the uptake' etc. We judge a person to be very intelligent, average or 'slow' on the basis of what they say and do – often by what they achieve in life. Intelligence itself cannot be seen, only the products of intelligence and these are very diverse. The world acknowledges that it takes a reasonable level of intelligence to compose a piece of music, write a novel, plan a battle, design a building, write a computer programme, manage a firm, navigate an aeroplane and so on. All of these activities are the products of intelligent minds, and parents and teachers judge a child to be intelligent or not by comparing him with other children in the family or at school.

Because intelligence is so important in life generally as well as in employment and in general education it has been studied intensely for many years and a very great body of knowledge relating to intelligence has been built up, but many of the findings have been challenged or contradicted and so the subject is a far from clear-cut one.

Some knowledge about how intelligence has been studied down the years may assist in understanding the situation.

1   In 1921 14 experts were asked to describe what they considered intelligence to be. The result of this was 14 different descriptions. However, there was a general agreement that intelligence involves:

(a) the capacity to learn from experience, and
(b) the ability to adapt to the surrounding environment.

2.   In 1927 it was proposed by Spearman that intelligence consists of two parts, or factors, one being a *general* factor and the other a *specific* factor. He proposed that there is only one general factor but many different specific factors. General ability is what we use when performing mental tasks of all kinds, and has been described as 'mental energy'. However, a specific ability is required for just one kind of mental task. Because of this it is possible for a person to be good at verbal skills (such as reading, writing and expressing themselves fluently in speech), good also at mathematics but to have little if any, musical ability and hence be quite poor when it comes to learning to play a musical instrument.

3.   In 1938 Thurstone argued that intelligence consists of a number of primary mental abilities which include verbal comprehension, word fluency, number, spatial visualisation, perceptual speed, memory and reasoning.

4.   In 1967 Guilford proposed that intelligence is made up of 120 elementary abilities.

5.   In 1971 Vernon proposed that intelligence can be described as comprising abilities at varying levels of generality. At the highest level is *general ability* (as proposed by Spearman), at the next level are '*major group factors*' (such as verbal-educational ability and practical-mechanical ability), below these are *minor group factors* and finally there are *specific factors* (as also proposed by Spearman).

6.   More recent work has attempted to prove that the different descriptions and definitions proposed in the past can be reduced to the same thing and a number of information-

processing psychologists have sought to understand general intelligence in terms of elementary components (or processes) used in the solution of various kinds of problems. They distinguish *meta-components* (used for planning), *acquisition components* (used in learning), *retention components* (used in remembering) *transfer components* (used in the transfer of knowledge from one task to another and *performance components* (used in the carrying out of a problem-solving strategy).

This information-processing view of intelligence seems to unify what were formally a number of differing views regarding the nature of intelligence.

However, a number of important questions relating to intelligence still remain to be answered. Three of these are:

• Is the meaning of 'intelligence' the same in all societies and different cultural groups?
• How accurately can intelligence tests predict the performance of people in the real world?
• Is intelligence largely inherited (as has been claimed by some) or is it largely, or even exclusively, determined by environment, as has been claimed by others?

One important fact that must be kept in mind when attempting to understand intelligence is that it is *not* a single, isolated entity (such as a person's height or weight) but is a *collection of abilities*, each one usually being the ability to reason in a particular way. Each one of us has all of these abilities but of course the *level* of each ability varies from one ability to another within each person. Because of this a person might be brilliant at maths and doing jigsaws but only moderate at writing a story and have almost no ability at all to paint a picture or play a musical instrument.

Not only is there variation within each person but there is also very wide variation between one person and another. A very intelligent person is one who has quite high abilities overall, an average person is one with moderate levels across the ability range and a slow learner has a low level of abilities overall. However, that is not to say that a highly intelligent person is very good at *everything*. In one or two areas of achievement such a person might have only a moderate, or even a poor, ability but nevertheless, when *all* abilities are considered, then he or she will be found to be quite high overall.

Intelligence can be better understood if we compare it with something such as *athleticism*. We all know what an athletic person is and can recognise them when we meet them. We also know how such a person differs from a non-athletic person. Nevertheless the concept is still vague rather than exact. If we consider a pentathlete, such a person needs to be very good at five different athletic activities. But it is possible for a number of people to take part in a pentathlon and for the overall winner not to be best at anything. A simple example should make this clear.

Imagine that six people compete in a pentathlon and end up with the places shown in Table 3.1. Remember that the competitor with the *lowest* total place score is the winner as the aim is to win five first places. (5 × 1 = 5) with the worst possible score to be five sixth places (5 × 6 = 30). As can be seen from the table, competitor A is the winner (and hence the most 'athletic' of the six who competed) yet did not come first in anything! He is considered the winner as he was sufficiently good *overall* to beat the other five *overall*. Each of the other five competitors was excellent at one event and proved it by coming first in the one event but proved not to be particularly good in most of the other events and so their average, and hence their overall result, came down below that of competitor A.

Table 3.1: Showing Places Gained by Six Competitors (A-F) in Pentathlon						
COMPETITORS						
EVENT	A	B	C	D	E	F
Riding	2	1st	6	4	5	3
Duelling	3	4	1st	5	6	2
Shooting	3	4	5	6	2	1st
Swimming	2	5	3	4	1st	6
Running	2	4	6	1st	5	3
Total of Places	12	18	21	20	19	15
Overall Position	1st	3	6	5	4	2

In just the same way the child who is considered to be 'top of the class' need not be the best in the class at every single subject taught. Likewise a highly intelligent person need not be excellent at everything and in fact might be quite poor at a few things in life. For the same reason a person considered to be 'average' or even generally 'slow' could well have one or two intellectual strengths, e.g. mental arithmetic.

The Assessment of Intelligence

For the best part of a century psychologists and others have been engaged in producing intelligence tests. Many have been produced and designed for different purposes, some for administering to whole groups at once, others to be administered to one person at a time, yet more intended for adults and a different set produced for use with children. Over time the process has become more refined and sophisticated. Some of the older ones have not withstood the test of time and have needed to be discarded, others have been periodically revised and updated; occasionally a new test is produced although, as will be explained later, they tend to be called SCALES nowadays.

The tests (or scales) attempt to assess an individual's potential to engage in purposive, useful behaviour, i.e. intelligent *activity*, rather than intelligence itself. Although there are many definitions of intelligence most of the tests/scales attempt to obtain an accurate picture of it by measuring a person's MENTAL ABILITIES or current INTELLECTUAL CAPACITIES.

The amount of agreement between experts on what it is that an intelligence test actually assesses is far greater than many people realise. An intelligence test is essentially a test of deductive reasoning and many psychologists prefer to talk of 'test of reasoning' than of 'intelligence'. More specific phrases are generally used, such as 'verbal reasoning', 'numerical reasoning', 'perceptual reasoning', etc. When a person's intelligence is measured by an intelligence test the result needs to be given in some form of measure or another. The INTELLIGENCE QUOTIENT (IQ for short) is the name given to the measure and we shall now see just what meaning there is in the figures given.

The IQ

When a test is administered to a child or indeed to any person the result is usually given as a number which is known as the intelligence quotient (IQ). There are a number of ways in which the result can be expressed but the IQ is the one most often used and certainly is the one best understood by the general population. However, improvements in the design of the tests mean that nowadays a lot more information is obtained about a child during the course of testing than can be conveyed by one simple number. In fact the question is often raised as to just what use an IQ figure is on its own. This is an important question because not only does the IQ not tell everything about a child's intellectual ability but under certain circumstances it may actually be misleading. How this can be so should become clear during the course of the chapter.

The manner in which intelligence tests are designed and the

means by which the IQ is derived from the test results are, in theory, quite logical and quite easy to understand.

Any test which is used consists of a number of items which are ranged in order from those considered to be very easy to those considered to be very difficult. The order of items is such that the difficulty increases in an orderly and gradual manner from one item to the other. (When we say 'item' we usually mean a question to be answered, an explanation given, a calculation to be made or a task to be completed).

The selection of items chosen will not have been assembled in any haphazard manner. Those used will usually have been the ones proven to be most appropriate from a much larger number. The order in which they have been arranged will also have been arrived at after much preliminary work in the form of 'pilot' studies. In the cases of tests designed for use with children two things are assumed. One is that any given child will be able to perform better on the same test as he gets older. (The seven-year-old child tested today will be able successfully to complete an even greater number of items in one year's time and more still a year after that).

The other is that any two children of the same age who are tested at the same time will achieve the *same* score if they are of EQUAL ABILITY. By the same token, if they are of *un*equal ability then they will obtain *different* scores, the more intelligent child being able to score higher than the less intelligent one. If the test does *not* do this - distinguish between children of different levels of intelligence - then it does not serve the purpose for which it was designed and will need to be abandoned.

Any properly designed test intended for use with children will have been piloted using large numbers of children spread through-out the age range for which the test is designed e.g. seven to sixteen years. By this means the basic design of the test will be effectively confirmed and the accuracy of the results derived will be checked and cross-checked. When this is completed it should be known exactly what score should be produced by an average seven-year-old, as well as an average child aged, say, 8;6 or 12;3.

Just like the reading test described in Chapter 1, an intelligence test can be viewed as a fairly long ladder reaching up from the ground with each rung marked as the natural stopping point for a normal child of a given age (see Fig. 1.5). In the case of a child aged eight he would be expected to 'climb the ladder' (so to speak) to the rung marked '8 yrs' and which would be higher than the '7 yrs' rung but below the '9 yrs' rung. What will be found in practice is that half of the eight-year-olds will be at or below this rung with the other half at or above it. Slower eight-year-olds will not be able to climb that far but brighter eight-year-olds will be able to climb above it. Some eight-year-olds will be on the '9 yrs' rung, a smaller number on the '10 yrs' rung and a very few even higher. Similarly some will occupy the '7 yrs' rung, some fewer the '6 yrs' one and a very few will be below this. The whole population of eight-year-old children, if tested, will be found to be spread across a range with the '8 yrs' rung marking the *average* stopping place for them. Most will be on either side of this rung or one within easy reach of it. Only small numbers are found at extremely high or extremely low positions.

Talking about rungs on ladders is all very well but it is not the easiest or the clearest way in which to give information about a child's intellectual abilities. The easiest way is actually by a scale of *numbers*, rather than ladder rungs and for this reason the system that has been used since the earliest days of intelligence testing has been to let the number 100 stand for AVERAGE INTELLIGENCE with other numbers spanning either side of it from 50 (or less) to 150 (or greater).

In fact, the scale is sometimes divided up into *sections* and sometimes also *descriptions* are used in order to make the IQ scores more meaningful. One scale ranges from 70 to 130 and has the divisions and descriptions as follows:

130 and above = very superior (or exceptionally high);
120–129 = superior (or high);
110–119 = bright average (or high average);
90–109 = average;
80–89 = low average;
70–79 = borderline (or low)
Below 70 = mentally retarded (or exceptionally low).

When the IQ scores of the population are used to produce a graph the result is as shown in Figure 3.1. As can be seen the average IQ for the population is 100. Most individuals lie between 85 and 115 (marked by dotted lines) and this is known as the normal range. In fact 68% of the total lies between these two IQ scores leaving 16% at the bottom end (below average) and the same percentage at the top. When a child is tested the score he obtains is compared with the *average* score for children of this age and by this means it is known whether he is average, above average, or below.

All that has been written so far could be applied quite simply if

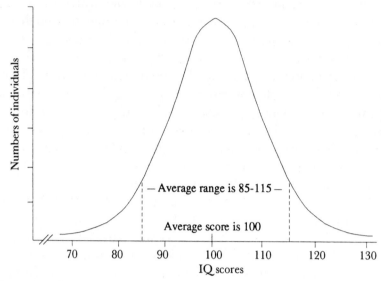

Figure 3.1 IQ scores of the UK's population

intelligence was known to be a *single* entity such as a person's height or weight. In that case it would be quite easy to assess a child's intelligence just by asking him a number of questions of increasing difficulty, finding out where the 'ceiling' of his ability was and then consulting a table to see how his score compared with most other children of the same age. In other words his single 'raw' score could be converted into a single 'scaled' score, from which his IQ would be known.

Unfortunately things are not quite that simple because, as was made clear earlier, intelligence is *not* considered to be a *single* ability but is instead a *collection* of abilities (just as 'athleticism' is a collection of abilities relating to a number of sporting events and not just one).

Therefore, to obtain an accurate picture of a child's intelligence it is necessary to test a *number* of the child's separate intellectual abilities and to see not only how they average out across the whole range but to observe what sort of a *pattern* or *'profile'* results from them.

The intelligence tests produced in recent years, and which are in general use by educational psychologists and others, all fit in with this basic design. Present-day intelligence tests are really collections of mini-tests (or sub-tests, to give them their correct name), each of which assesses something different about the child's ability to reason, solve problems and manipulate concepts etc.

The question arises as to just what abilities an intelligence test should be designed to assess. After all, people possess a wide range of abilities. (Remember that Guilford claimed that intelligence is made up of 120 different mental abilities). It would be impossible to test all of them. Whatever number is chosen it must be a reasonably small one as there are advantages in having a test that requires a reasonably small amount of equipment (for easy transportation from school to school etc.) and can be administered within a reasonable period of time (1 hour seems to be the most common time for this).

The abilities tested tend to be selected by the test designers on the basis of those which best represent GENERAL INTELLIGENCE as it is thought that these

- produce the greatest information about a child's mental capacity;
- act as useful tools in the field of educational assessment;
- help to appraise learning and other disabilities;
- can be used to predict future school performance accurately.

The Wechsler Intelligence Scale for Children (WISC)

This test (or rather scale) needs to be described and its results interpreted for a number of reasons. First, it is a well-established scale whose design is very helpful in assessing children's learning difficulties. It has also undergone a number of revisions since it was first produced. The WISC is probably the most commonly used of all the tests/scales available to educational psychologists and is certainly a very popular one with them.

Second, the WISC is designed to be used in children aged from seven to sixteen years of age and thus covers almost the entire age range of the school population in the British Isles. There are companion scales to the WISC which are a downward extension (the WPPSI) and an upward extension (the WAIS) and so younger or older pupils may be assessed by means of these if required.

This is probably a good point at which to explain why the word 'test' is no longer officially used and has been replaced by 'scale'. A *test* is something which a person either *passes* or *fails*. (The driving test is a good example of this.) With intelligence testing, however, it is *not* a question of 'pass' or 'fail', but simply a question of obtaining a *measure* and so the WISC and other similar instruments should be regarded as a scale or measure by which the child is compared with others of the same age. It is more like a ruler or a pair of bathroom scales. However, despite these changes the expression 'intelligence test' is very much a part of everyday speech and will be used in this book from time to time.

To return to our description of the WISC, it has been designed and organised to measure *general intelligence*. The particular sub-tests used in the WISC were selected on the basis of two concepts:

(a)   that intelligence is an overall or global entity which is multi-determined and multi-factored *rather* than an independent, uniquely-defined trait;

(b)   that no one particular ability is of any very great importance compared with any other.

The WISC consists of a number of sub-tests which are divided into two groups:
the VERBAL sub-tests and
the PERFORMANCE sub-tests.

It is possible for a psychologist to administer to the child:

• the VERBAL sub-tests only and hence derive a VERBAL IQ,

or   • the PERFORMANCE sub-tests only and hence derive a PERFORMANCE IQ,

or   • BOTH sets of sub-tests and hence derive a FULL-SCALE IQ.

The Verbal Scale

This consists of six sub-tests but normally only five of them are administered to the child as the results from five are adequate to produce a reliable verbal IQ. The sixth sub-test is available to the psychologist as a supplementary sub-test, to be used in the event of one of the others being spoiled. However, it can also be administered in order to yield useful information in its own right. The verbal sub-tests are:

•   Information
•   Similarities
•   Arithmetic
•   Vocabulary
•   Comprehension
•   (Digit Span - the supplementary test).

The Performance Scale

This also consists of six sub-tests, only five of which are usually administered. The performance sub-tests are:

- Picture Completion
- Picture Arrangement
- Block Design
- Object Assembly
- Coding
- (Mazes – the supplementary test).

The scaled scores which children can obtain on the sub-tests range from 1 to 19, the average score of each being 10 and most scores grouped around this from 8 to 12.

Much will become clearer if we take the scores of an imaginary average child (whom we will call child A). Such a child could well obtain a set of scaled scores as set out in Table 3.2

Table 3.2:		SCORES OF CHILD A	
VERBAL		PERFORMANCE	
Information	11	Picture Completion	12
Similarities	8	Picture Arrangement	10
Arithmetic	10	Block Design	8
Vocabulary	9	Object Assembly	9
Comprehension	10	Coding	11

An instant 'picture' or profile of child A's intelligence is given to us by the graph which can be produced from his scores. (The WISC/R-S test form on which the child's results are written is provided with a grid for this very purpose). Child A's graph is shown in Figure 3.2.

A number of features can be noted:

- The verbal scores add up to 48 which converts (by means of a special set of tables) into a *verbal IQ* of 97.
- Likewise, the performance scores add up to 50 and convert into a *performance IQ* of 100.
- The total of totals of the verbal tests (48) and performance tests (50) themselves add together to make 98 which can also be converted into a *full-scale IQ* of 98.
- Child A is, therefore, of average range overall ability as he lies within the IQ range of 85 to 115. What is more, he is only 2 points different from the mean of 100.
- The full-scale or overall IQ of 98 was obtained from combining a verbal IQ of 97 and a performance IQ of 100. These two IQs (97 and 100) are very close to one another, the difference

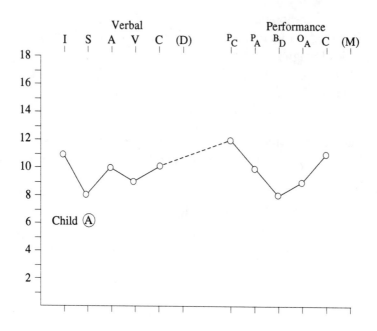

Figure 3.2 WISC scores of average ability (child A)

being only 3. This is the situation as shown by most children. A difference of just a few points is quite common and large differences are quite rare. For example, a difference of 12 points between verbal and performance IQs is found only five times in a hundred by chance alone. If there is a difference of 12 points within an individual child there are only five chances in 100 that the difference has occurred by chance alone and 95 chances in 100 that something has *caused* it. Even larger differences than 12 are found in ever smaller percentages of children with very large differences being very rare indeed.

•   The five verbal scores are tightly 'banded' together as the lowest is 8 and the highest 11 and so are separated by only 3 points. Because of this the profile of the verbal scale of the graph is quite 'flat' or 'even' with no extremes, i.e. no very high 'peaks' or very deep 'valleys'.

•   The same applies to the performance items.

We can now compare these findings with those of another child – one of low ability whom we will call child L. Imagine that he has produced the scores given in Table 3.3. The graph produced by these scores in shown in Figure 3.3.

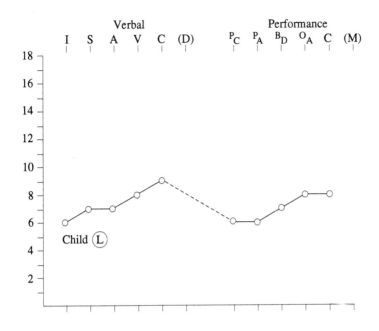

Figure 3.3 WISC scores of low ability (child L)

Table 3.3		
Verbal Scores	6, 7, 7, 8, 9 Total = 37	*Verbal IQ = 85*
Performance Scores	6, 6, 7, 8, 8 Total = 35	*Performance IQ = 80*
		Full-Scale IQ = 80

As can be seen, the verbal scores and the performance scores are all low as even the highest (9) is below the population average of 10. The verbal scores total to only 37 which convert to a verbal IQ of 85, the average for the population being 100. In the same way the performance tests produce a total of only 35 and a performance IQ of 80.

The verbal and performance score totals (37 and 35) when added together produce 72 which converts to a full-scale IQ of 80. A score of 80 or less applies to the least gifted 9% of the total population.

However, each set of scores is, once again, quite tightly 'banded' together (between 6 and 9 in the case of the verbal scores and between 6 and 8 with the performance ones). No *large* variations are found and this is the case with the vast majority of children, whether they are of high, average or low intelligence. With child L the *general* picture is exactly the same as that of child A except that the scores lie lower down the graph.

The last part of the overall picture is obtained by considering a child of high ability – child H. The scores for this fictitious child are given in Table 3.4.

Table 3.4:		
Verbal Scores	13, 14, 12,13,14 Total = 66	*Verbal IQ = 119*
Performance Scores	15,12,13,14,12 Total = 66	*Performance IQ = 122*
		Full-Scale IQ = 122

When we analyse these figures we see that the same picture emerges as in child A and child L except that the graph which results will lie higher up the paper. We can see this for ourselves by looking at the next illustration (Figure 3.4), which consists of the graphs of the three children displayed on the same axes or framework.

The child of high ability lies above the average child who is, in turn, above the child of low ability. The three graphs are all more or less the same as one another, being quite 'flat' in each case, i.e. showing only a small range in the spread of scores.

When educational psychologists assess children they are particularly interested in children who show themselves to be different from the majority. It is possible for the graph of a child's WISC scores to show one of two types of difference. The first is for the verbal and performance scores to be at different levels, *either* the verbal being at

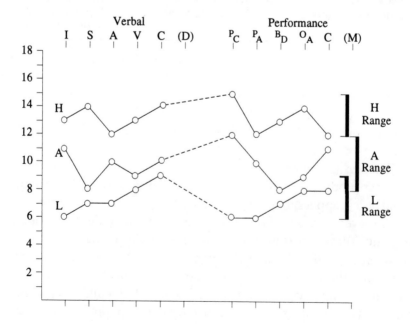

Figure 3.4 High, average and low ability children displayed together for comparison

a high level and the performance at a low level *or* the other way round. When this is found then an explanation for it must be sought, usually by further investigation. However, in many such cases it is unlikely to have any bearing on the subject of dyslexia.

The other type of variation is for the graph not to be very even but instead to show a wide range of scores, producing quite marked 'peaks' and 'valleys'. It is considered by many that this second type of graph can indicate dyslexia, particularly if certain sub-tests are at the low points. The particular sub-tests concerned are Information, Arithmetic, Digit span and Coding. If the initials of these are taken and their order is rearranged the word 'ACID' is formed which, in the circumstances, is thought by many to be very appropriate as it allows them to talk about the *'Acid' tests* that can indicate dyslexia.

This type of graph shape or profile is shown in Figure 3.5.

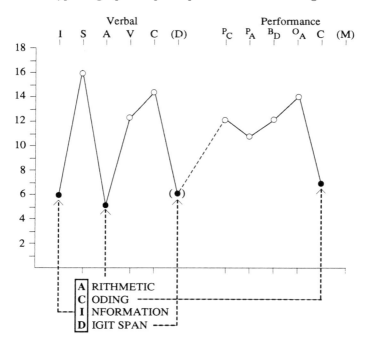

Figure 3.5 A possible profile of a dyslexic child (note the 'ACID' tests)

Before we end this chapter a word of explanation about the WISC is required. The WISC has existed in three forms: that is to say the original version has been updated twice. The information in this chapter is based on the WISC-R[s] which is the second version (first up-dating) and which became available in 1978. (The 'R' stands for Revised and the 'S' for Scottish norms). Since then – in 1992 – the third version (second revision) has become available and is the

WISC-III[UK] (the UK stands for the fact that norms based on a population in the United Kingdom have been obtained and are used with children tested in the UK).

Over time the WISC III[UK] will replace the WISC-R[S] and parents will be more likely to find that this is the test (or scale) being used by educational psychologists and being quoted in their reports. However, none of the 11 sub-scales described in this chapter has been replaced and so the use of the WISC-III[UK] instead of the WISC-R[S] will make no difference to the outcome. Now that we have discussed the important part played by intelligence we need to find out about its connection with mental age as this has a large part to play in the diagnosis of dyslexia. Mental age is explained in the next chapter.

Chapter 4:
The Importance of
Mental Age

The earlier chapters covered some important ground which we need to understand in order to appreciate the problems met in connection with dyslexia. We now know that we need to be able to measure a child's reading ability accurately and objectively. We also know that reading ability is measured in terms of reading age and that a child's reading age can be obtained only by the use of an accurately designed and well-standardised reading test. We have dealt with the fact that any group of similarly aged children will between them show variations in reading age (assuming that the group have not been previously selected on the basis of reading age). Some will be different from average – either above or below it – with half of these in each group. Because of this, when we are considering a child who is suspected of being dyslexic it could well be difficult if not impossible for us to decide whether he is dyslexic or not unless we can *prove* in some way that:

- the child is reading less well than he should;
- his difficulty is due to dyslexia and *not* some other reason.

After all, the mere fact that the child is reading less well than other children of the same age is not *on its own* a sufficient reason to suspect that dyslexia is present. In the first place he could be of low intelligence and so belong naturally, so to speak, to that group of backward readers – the bottom 15% or so. Second, as will become clear eventually, it is possible for a child to have an *average* reading age and *still* be affected by dyslexia. There will be good grounds for suspecting dyslexia is part of the picture only if it can be shown that he is basically capable of achieving better and would be doing so if he were not dyslexic. At this point we are left with an all-important question:

> Is there any way we can calculate how well a child can be EXPECTED to read – as opposed to how well he actually does read – and, if so, how can this be done?

Fortunately we *can* do this, by making use of the idea of a person's MENTAL AGE. Mental age can be calculated quite simply. What mental age is, the reason why we can use it, and the way in which it is calculated can be understood if we first compare the *intelligence test scores* produced by a group of children with the *reading ages* that they have achieved.

Let us take as an example a large group of ten-year-olds. We need to consider thousands rather than hundreds and we need to choose them on a completely random basis, not by any kind of deliberate selective process. In short, we want our group to be truly representative of the whole population of ten-year-olds in the country and to be in effect a 'scale model' of the total. (We have selected the ten-year-olds as it makes the calculations that need to be done easier than otherwise, but what we say applies equally well to *any* group of school-age children.

When the IQs produced by the group are set out in the form of a graph, the result is as in Figure 4.1.

When the *same* ten-year-olds each have their reading progress tested and their reading ages are produced as a graph the result is as in Figure 4.2.

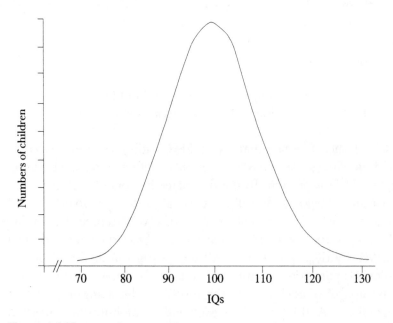

Figure 4.1 IQ scores of ten-year-olds

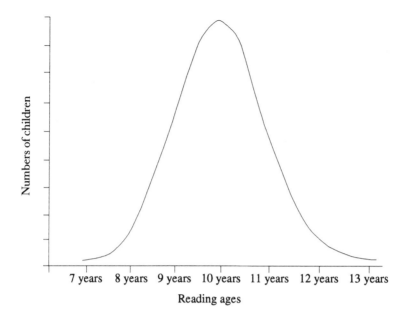

Figure 4.2 Reading ages of ten-year-olds

Obviously the graphs are identical. Our large group of children have been assessed on two aspects of their development – intelligence and reading ability – and have produced overall results on one which *match* the overall results of the other. The children have been found to be a mixture of low, average and high intelligence. They are also a mixture of poor, average and good readers.

Because there is such a close match of the *overall* results it is tempting to assume that there is individual matching – a situation of very close correlation. That is to say, we are tempted into thinking that the children who have the high intelligence are the same ones who have the good reading ages, that average IQ is linked with average reading ability and low IQ with poor reading. But this is an assumption which at this stage we are not allowed to make, tempting though it might be. We need *proof*, and without it can go no further.

Proof is vital. The fact of the matter is that the graphs produced by intelligence and reading age when quite large numbers of children are measured are exactly the same shape as *many other* aspects of human development. Graphs of this shape are quite common and the shape itself is known as 'the normal curve'. Height and weight are two other aspects of children which would produce the same shape of graph if a sufficiently large number of them were measured.

If, instead of intelligence, the height of each ten-year-old had been measured and a graph drawn we would have found it to be of similar shape to that produced by intelligence. We then would have had a situation such that the graphs of height and reading age of the large groups of ten-year-olds were found to be a match for one another. However, that would not entitle us to assume that tall children were better readers than average-size children nor that average size ones were better than small ones. No correlation between height and reading ability has ever been shown.

Further investigation and information is required. However, when we make it we are rewarded because our assumption turns out to be *true!*

Children with high IQs *are* found to be the same children who have high reading ages. Children with high IQs do not fall into groups of good, average and poor readers but stay concentrated at the 'good' end of the distribution of reading ages. This is what we discover when detailed comparisons are made. In the same way those children of average intelligence produce average reading ages and those of low-range IQs have poor reading ages also. These findings might be obvious and, it could be claimed, were predictable, but that is not the point. What is of importance is that we have been able to move past the point of guesswork and now have the knowledge we need to be able to move forward with certainty.

The situation can be illustrated as in Figure 4.3. In by far the majority of cases, therefore, intelligence is a good *predictor* of reading age. It can be, and is, used as a means of calculating what any particular child's reading age should be. When we compare intelligence with reading we need to remember that intelligence as we refer to it is a *general* ability but that reading is a highly *specific* skill.

Because of the nature of intelligence we find that it acts as a good *predictor* of how well a child should be performing in school subjects generally – those with an academic content, that is. We are talking about those in which success depends on the ability to remember, discover relationships, perform calculations, and benefit from past experiences, etc.

What teachers and others working with children have come to find useful is the idea that each child possesses a certain MENTAL AGE. A child's mental age can be calculated from his intelligence and can then be used to predict his reading age.

The idea on which mental age is based is that any child of *average* intelligence has a mental age that is *equal* to the child's chronological age, but if his intelligence is higher then his mental age will be greater. Naturally it follows that if the child is of low intelligence his

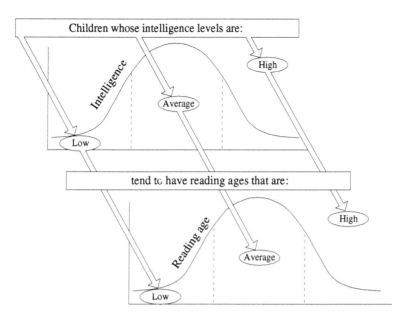

Figure 4.3 The relationship between intelligence and reading age

mental age will be less than his chronological age.

Mental age can be thought of as a measure of how much the child's general mental abilities have been able to develop during his lifetime. Although it is quite adequate for certain purposes to know that a child is of average, high or low ability, for other circumstances this is not accurate enough. Often it is necessary to know more than in which particular one of these three categories the child happens to belong.

It is possible for a child to be described as 'average' and for that child to have an IQ as low as 85 which means that he is more able than 17% of the population. But is also possible for another child to be described as 'average' and for this one to have an IQ as high as 115 which makes him more able than 83% of the population. The term 'average' covers quite a wide range indeed and to have two children such as the ones just described both to be termed 'average' can lead to confusion.

Mental age is a vast improvement on this system as it is an *exact* measure and is given in years and months just as is a child's chronological age. In order to calculate Mental Age all that needs to be known is a child's age and IQ. The calculation is quite simple:

(i)   The chronological age (CA) and IQ are multiplied together (CA x IQ).

(ii)   The number which results is then divided by 100.

$$\frac{(CA \times IQ)}{100}$$

This is the child's mental age (MA). In other words:

$$MA = \frac{(CA \times IQ)}{100}$$

For example, in the case of a child who is aged exactly ten (CA = 10 yrs) and whose IQ is 80, his mental age (MA) will be 8 yrs.

$$MA = \frac{(10 \times 80)}{100} \text{ yrs}$$

$$MA = \frac{800}{100} \text{ yrs}$$

$$MA = 8 \text{ yrs}$$

In exactly the same way a child aged 10 and with an IQ of 125 will have a mental age of 12 ½ yrs.

$$MA = \frac{(10 \times 125)}{100} \text{ yrs}$$

$$MA = 12 \text{ ½ yrs } (or \ 12;6)$$

In the case of the first child, because his IQ is 80 (which is 20 below the average of 100) it is considered that throughout each year of his life he has been able to learn at a slower rate than normal – at 80% or ⅘ of the normal rate, in fact. Hence at the age of 10 years, it is considered that he has been only able to gain the same amount of general knowledge and learning experience as an average eight-year-old, and so this is his mental age.

The second child, on the other hand, has been sufficiently intelligent as to be able to learn at about one and a quarter times the normal rate (1¼ or 1.25 or 125% of normal) and so at the age of ten he has acquired the same amount of knowledge, experience and understanding as an average child aged 12;6.

Having moved from the position of knowing the child's age and IQ to calculating his mental age, how do we move from there to finding his expected reading age? Quite simply, *mental age and expected reading age always have the same value.* Whatever mental age a child happens to have his reading age can be *expected* to match it. A child with a mental age of 8 years should be able to read at the 8 yrs level (as well as perform at the 8 years level in other tasks and skills). Someone with a mental age of 11 years should have a reading age of 11 years also. The whole procedure can be summarised as:

$$\frac{(CA \times IQ)}{100}$$ will give *mental age* which is the same as *expected reading age*

For a group of children who are all of the same age (CA) it is possible to link IQ, mental age (MA) and expected reading age (expected RA) together by means of a simple diagram. All three of these are interconnected in a straightforward and easily understood manner and so each can be represented by a 'ladder' with it being possible to set the three 'ladders' side by side. In the case of any given child, when his position on the first 'ladder' is located then his position on any of the other two is determined by a simple move sideways, always staying at the same height whatever 'ladder' the child is on. This is made clearer by Figure 4.4. Once again we have chosen the age of 10 as an example so as to make calculating easier but the same rules apply *whatever* the child's age.

We are now in a position to appreciate exactly what information is necessary before it can be said with any certainty that a child *could* possibly be dyslexic – let alone definitely is so.

A dyslexic child must always have an *actual* reading age which is *lower* than his *expected* reading age. It is not sufficient to suspect dyslexia merely on the basis of a child's reading being below average because such a child could be of low intelligence and hence not be able to produce any better results. This is a case of a *general* learning difficulty and such a child is described as a backward reader, as we have made clear earlier.

Where dyslexia is concerned we are dealing with a *specific* learning difficulty. The child's general level of intelligence allows his expected reading age to be calculated and his actual reading age must be found to be below this. What we are doing, in fact, is comparing the child who is suspected of being dyslexic with all other children who are of the *same age and of the same level of intelligence* as himself. In other words we are comparing him with all other children of the *same MENTAL AGE*. If his reading age is less than it should be on *this* basis then we have a retarded reader, not a backward one, and dyslexia *might* be the cause of the retardation.

When a shortfall is discovered between his expected and actual

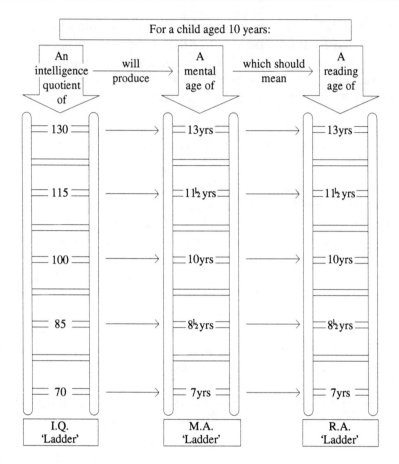

Figure 4.4

reading ages we are only at the first stage of the process. It is possible for the depressed reading age to be accounted for by visual difficulties, hearing problems or indeed any of the many possible causes listed in the previous chapter. It is only when these can be discounted as possible causes that we are entitled to claim that dyslexia or specific learning difficulties is likely as the explanation.

Summary

1. When a child's reading age is below average it is possible for this to be due to one of two reasons, *backwardness* or *retardation.*
2. Without further investigation it is not possible to know to which of these two very different categories the child belongs. A *backward* reader has difficulties owing to lack of basic ability to do any better. Half of all children will be below average but

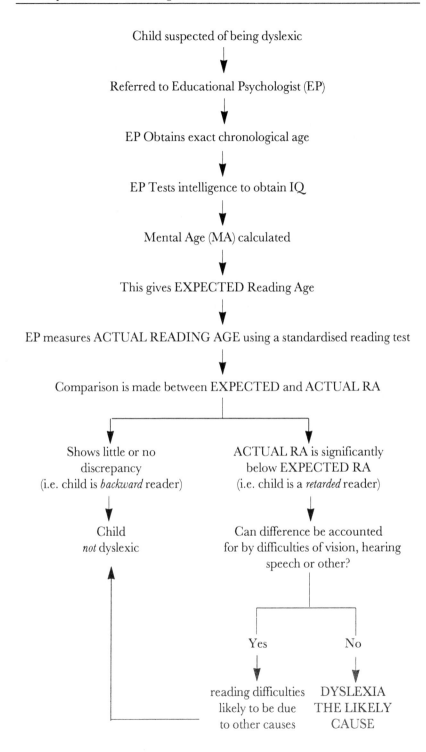

Figure 4.5: Steps in the investigation of suspected dyslexia

it is usually the worst 17% or so that are considered to be backward.

A *retarded* reader does possess the basic ability to read better but is being held back (or retarded) by one or more influences. Dyslexic children are part of this group but not all retarded readers are dyslexic as a child's retardation could be due to other reasons.

3.   The way to investigate whether a child is backward or retarded is to calculate what his expected reading age is and compare this with his *actual* reading age.

4.   The expected reading age is the same as mental age which can be calculated from the child's exact chronological age and his IQ.

5.   In this way, by knowing the child's exact age, IQ and actual reading age any shortfall or discrepancy can be uncovered.

6.   Such a discrepancy is only an indication that dyslexia *could* be the cause. Further investigation will then be required in order to exclude other possible causes.

The procedure is summarised in Figure 4.5.

Chapter 5:
The Teaching of
Reading

Reading involves the bringing together and mastery of a number of skills. Reading is preceded by the development of speech which is, in turn, just one of the many forms of communication, all of which are made possible through and generated by means of man's intelligence. We can represent this in a simple diagram (see Figure 5.1).

Although the use of language is a natural attribute of man, the ability to read is an acquired skill. In fact it represents the acquisition of a number of sub-skills (most of them quite complex) and involves the essential knack of learning to get them all together and to use them in an automatic, almost effortless manner.

The manner in which children learn to read is largely still a mystery to us, but the skills they need to master and the knowledge

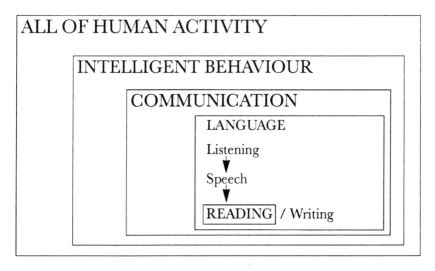

Figure 5.1

they need to acquire is quite well known and easily described. *What* children *experience* in the various stages through which they must pass, from being quite illiterate to fully literate has been recorded in quite full details but exactly *how* it is done is still largely unknown. We do not understand the neuro-psychology involved but we do know that for most children all they require is the proper opportunity and the proper encouragement right at the start and in the early stages

In learning to read children enter a world that is new to them, full of rules which are often quite arbitrary and sometimes completely contradictory. It is stating the obvious, of course, to say that in our society children learn to read mainly from books. When quite young they need to know that books contain words and so are important in reading, that they open at the right-hand side and have a 'spine' on the left, that a book consists of sheets of paper called pages, that each page has a 'top' (the edge furthest away) and a 'bottom' (the edge closest to the reader), a left side and a right side.

Children need to know that the marks (usually coloured black) on the pages (usually coloured white) consist of print and that the print tells the story. They must learn that the printed story is set out in straight lines and that these lines, in our culture, are arranged from the top of the page to the bottom, one after the other with each individual line running from left to right and hence needing to be read that way. Reading a line of print the way we do, moving our eyes steadily from left to right in small jerky movements is, in fact, a quite unnatural way of looking at anything. Normally our eyes do not move in this way. (Some cultures read lines of writing from right to left, others write in columns of letters *down* the page.)

The learning process must continue on to master the fact that a line of print consists of words, each word being made up of a collection of letters in a certain order with white spaces being left between each word

asdoingitthatwaymakesitmucheasiertoreadandunderstand

and there will also be small spaces left between letters of a word. This is done not only to print in books

but also when we do handwriting like this although not when we are using this style, usually known as "double writing"

All this, of course, is only the beginning. The 26 letters of the alphabet, of which all of our written words are composed, can each be found in two sizes:

CAPITAL (ALSO KNOWN AS UPPER-CASE) SIZE, and

small (also known as lower-case) size.

What is more confusing is that although eight of the letters are identical in both capital and small form (Cc – Oo – Ss – Uu – Vv – Ww – Xx – Zz) the majority are quite different (Aa – Bb – Dd – Ee – etc.). A few letters can appear in different printed shapes when in the lower case form (for example a ɑ – g ɡ – q ɋ). The confusion continues when the child who is beginning to read has to learn to differentiate between pairs of letters that are mirror-images of each other, or virtually so (bd – pq – mw – un) and also needs to be sufficiently alert not to confuse the small L (written as l) with the capital i (written as I).

As most children are building up their number skills at the same time as they are learning to read, this fact can also lead to many confusions. The *number* 0 which we call 'nought' or 'zero' can be confused with the *letter* O; similarly the number 1 (one) can be confused with the lower case L (l) or the capital i (I), 2 and 5 can be confused with the letter S, 6 with the letters b or d and 9 with the letters g, p or q.

The Teaching of Reading in Schools

Reading has been taught in the British Isles in a widespread, regular and systematic manner for well over 120 years – since the Education Act of 1870, in fact. Although before 1870 many were taught reading these tended to be children of the well-to-do who were themselves literate, wanted their children to be likewise, and had the money available to spend on their education. From 1870 onwards education became widespread and all children were supposed to attend school regularly, so that reading, writing and arithmetic (the 3 Rs) could be learned by them along with a number of other basic subjects and educational skills.

The teaching of reading has undergone a process of great change during the period of 120 and more years that all children in the British Isles have been required to attend school and hence be taught. Most of the changes have been as a result of advances in knowledge relating to how children learn, the various factors concerned with learning (such as motivation, attention, memory etc.) and the processes involved in child development. As a result there has been an increase in awareness of types of difficulties that are likely to arise in a child when attempting to master the skill of reading.

Teaching styles vary tremendously and the conditions under which children are taught can also vary a great deal, but throughout the past 120 or so years teaching approaches have tended to follow a certain pattern.

Originally a child was taught to read by using just *one book* – and this tended to be the Bible. Over time various teachers who were also writers produced *sets of reading books*, graded from simple to more complex. Today most children are taught by means of *reading schemes* and these, interestingly enough, tend to be produced by publishing firms rather than individual writers. Well-known names in this branch of publishing are GINN 360 and LADYBIRD. (We shall be saying more about reading schemes later on.) At the present time it is true to say that there is no single absolutely correct and perfect way to teach a child to read. Methods which one teacher finds quite successful will be found to work badly with another teacher. Also, the same teacher encountering two different classes of children will find that what works well with the first class will not be as successful with the second. This is because the process of learning to read is a very *complex mixture* of the skills, talents, abilities and personality factors etc. which were referred to earlier. What usually happens is that a teacher works by bringing together her knowledge of the individual children and also a knowledge of the various techniques of teaching (including the strengths and weaknesses of each technique).

Whenever the techniques of teaching reading are described they are usually divided into two main methods which are:

(i)   THE 'WHOLE' METHOD (or 'LOOK and SAY' approach);
(ii)   THE PHONIC METHOD (or 'sounding-out' approach).

At certain stages in the history of education some methods have gained a special prominence for a period of time but this is usually some time after the theories on which they were based were first put forward. Teachers tend to be conservative in their approaches and hence unlikely to change techniques at short notice.

It is usually found that teachers gradually adopt a new approach by trying it out and then using it more and more, slowly dropping what they were using previously. One writer has described this as a 'grafting-on' process. As a result most teachers will be found not to be using entirely a 'whole' method nor entirely a 'phonic' method but generally a mixture of both.

Whole-word methods

(a) *The Story Method*: Some reading schemes were based on repetition and memorisation of stories and, as is only to be expected, were later criticised as teaching children to learn the contents of a book by heart rather than by reading it. However, despite its limitations, children did learn to read by this method and so it had at least some factors in its favour. The children enjoyed the rhythm and the repetition involved and of course the method is still used by teachers with material such as nursery rhymes, as well by parents in the home.

(b) *Word Patterns*: This was a method of teaching reading by getting the child to look on each word as a particular *shape* or pattern, rather than as a number of letters placed in a certain order. Interest grew after Helen Davidson published research in 1931 and the method was strongly associated with Gates, an American.

Words are considered to occupy certain shapes, as in Figure 5.2.

By this method children could build up to a stage where they were able to read sentences without realising that words were made up of letters.

The later stages of Davidson's work were used far more than the former ones and the 'look and say' method developed as a result, but in a form where actual words are used from the very

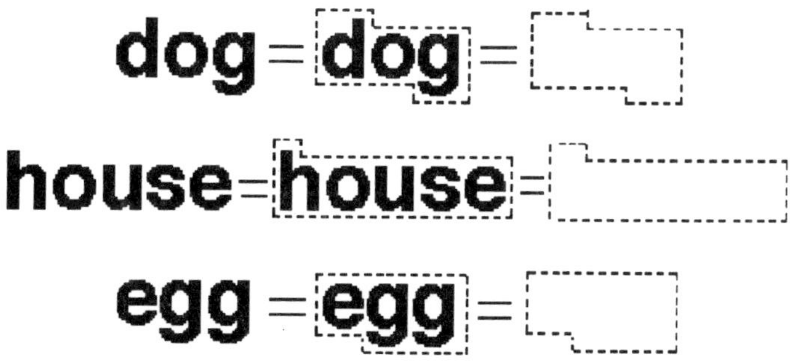

Figure 5.2

beginning, the words being taught by the use of pictures, flash cards etc.

The method became very popular in the 1940s and many schools dropped the 'phonic drill' technique which they had used previously. Many authorities on the teaching of reading since then have recommended that the 'look and say' approach should be used exclusively in the early stages of reading growth.

(c) *Kinaesthetic Method*: In 1921 Fernand and Kelly formulated the Kinaesthetic method in America. As normal schools taught reading using predominantly visual and auditory approaches Fernand investigated whether the *sense of touch* could be used to teach reading to children who had previously failed.

In this method the child traced over a word which had been written in cursive (i.e. 'double') writing on a piece of card, the word being spoken aloud as the tracing commenced. The tracing was continued until the word could be produced from memory. Many words were learned in this way, after which the writing of words was attempted, and later still, sentences. With certain children there was great success but with others there was complete failure. However the approach did emphasise the importance of introducing writing at the same time as reading, as well as highlighting the importance of establishing good 'left-to-right' orientation in children learning to read.

(d) *The Sentence Method*: This became popular in 1929 when Jagger (a London inspector of schools) published his book *The Sentence Method of Teaching Reading*, but the idea had been around since the end of the nineteenth century.

In this method children are shown a picture and the teacher and children discuss it. The children compose their own sentences and certain of these are selected and written beneath the picture. When a sentence can be read fluently with the picture present the child attempts to match it with an identical sentence and then read it *without* the picture as a guide. When a number of sentences have become very familiar to the child he can then be expected to recognise individual words from them. At a later stage books are introduced.

This method has much to recommend it as it is a child-centred one, with the child providing his own reading matter out of his own personal experiences and so reading only sentences he himself has composed. Reading is thereby meaningful and is contained within the child's own language ability.

Phonic methods

(a)   *Alphabetic Method*: In this the child was taught to recognise each letter of the alphabet in turn by its name. With each new word the child met he had to read out the name of each letter in the word and then say the word itself. (For example, the word *hat* would produce the response 'aitch-ay-tee-hat'). It was *thought* that by working in this way the child would look so carefully at the printed word that he would not only learn to read but to spell also.

   The Alphabetic method was criticised quite strongly. Although the child received a great deal of practice in letter recognition and left-to-right movement of the eye along each letter and line of print, on the other hand the fluency of reading was held back and at the same time the child was not given any assistance in working out how any printed word was pronounced.

   However, the Alphabetic method did achieve demands for a reform of the spelling system.

(b)   *Diacritical Marks*: The 26 symbols we know as the letters of the alphabet have been replaced by different people at different times in an attempt to make the process of learning to read easier.

   Gattegno used 41 colours in his scheme, entitled 'Words in Colour'.

   The Initial Teaching Alphabet (ITA) used 44 symbols but the diacritical system (which was designed by Richard and Maria Edgeworth in 1798) used 73 different symbols. Marks were used to indicate different sounds of a letter.

   The obvious criticism of this system was that it was more difficult for a child to learn 73 symbols than only 26 and the amount of decoding which the child would have had to do would have been excessive. Other similar systems have been designed over the years but there has never been a great following for any of them.

(c)   *The Work of Nellie Dale*: This lady is often credited with having invented the phonic method of teaching reading. However, what she produced was a combination of certain earlier experiences with two new ideas of her own.

   The first of these was her insistence upon ear, hand and eye training. The second was the use of colour as an aid (early on in the teaching process) to the recognition of the sound value of letters, e.g. red print for vowels and yellow print for silent letters. Only four colours were used in all and were introduced one at a time. However, in common with all other systems Ms Dale's method had its limitations.

The phonic approach, which had originally dominated the education system, found that it was being challenged first by the 'look and say', and later by the 'sentence' methods, so that during the 1930s and 40s it became relegated to second favourite.

The two main systems have long been in competition with one another and the results of research are far from clear-cut. Children learn to read at different speeds and also perhaps in different ways, however slight, from one individual to another, depending on each child's abilities, skills, interests and degree of motivation.

Most teachers, it is claimed, follow either one or the other method, but it is seen that in practice the situation tends not to be as clear-cut as is often thought. Those teachers who favour the *'look and say'* method believe that children learn to read more easily if they are presented repeatedly with a set number of words so that they eventually learn to recognise each one of them. This provides them with what is known as a basic 'sight vocabulary' which will continue to grow and from which they will learn the basic rules by which the 'code' of reading is 'cracked'.

Those teachers who favour the *Phonic* approach hold that children are best taught to read by having them first learn how to break down a printed word into its component *sounds* (known as phonemes) and then building up the phonemes into the complete sound of the word. With practice the process becomes quicker and smoother. By this means the printed word *cat* is sound out by the child as 'kerr-ah-tuh' and these three sounds are then blended together to make the sound of the spoken word 'cat'. In the same way *sun* is broken down to 'sss-uh-neh', to be blended into 'sun'.

Irrespective of whether the Look and Say or the Phonics approach is employed, almost all teachers make use of many of the same techniques and aids to literacy. In the past, much teaching of reading was achieved by means of set drills and exercises but in recent years reading has come to be considered as only one aspect of a language programme and hence *meaningful* reading is considered to be the all-important goal to be achieved.

Reading (and writing also) is found to be mastered most effectively by children if it is allowed to develop from their natural interests and activities. Pre-reading skills will be first established by encouraging the young child in the activities of listening and speaking, reading and writing. This will involve almost any mentally stimulating activity you can imagine: telling stories, looking at pictures, saying rhymes and jingles, singing songs, watching suitable television programmes, making use of the radio, playing with sand/water/ Plasticine etc., dressing up, acting out a play, using desk-top games such as dominoes, draughts, snakes and ladders etc., playing card games such as 'snap', sorting objects by size, by shape, by colour etc., doing jigsaws, playing with construction toys, playing on large apparatus such as the see-saw, swings, monkey-ladder, slide, climbing frame etc. All of these activities will encourage children to listen carefully, to take note of the details of things, to remember them and also to be able to speak about them.

The activity of reading proper is introduced to the child by such means as picture books and comics, road signs, flash cards, labels, notices, charts and other display material as well as the book corner of the classroom. Early on, children make books for themselves.

At the same time writing is introduced by such activities as scribbling, finger-painting, brush painting, pattern making, drawing a story in pictures, tracing pictures, tracing letters, joining lines by dot-to-dot, the drawing of circles and lines (the basic shapes and marks that go to make up lower-case letters) etc.

The intention lying behind the use of such teaching techniques is to develop skills such as *recognition, recall* and *discrimination*. For instance, the letter 'a' needs to be recognised whenever it is found in print. It may be found on its own (*a* pen), in a short word (h*a*t) or in a longer word (thous*a*nd). The sound which the letter 'a' makes needs to be *recalled* accurately on each occasion it appears. In reading it is vital for the child to be able to *discriminate* between one letter and another: 'a' is similar in appearance to c, e, o, u as each of them is small and rounded in appearance. Discrimination is particularly important in the case of those letters which have other letters as their mirror images and can thereby be even more easily confused (b and d/m and w/u and n/p and q).

The first word which a teacher introduces to a child tends to be the child's own name. Building on the child's immediate environment and interests usually results in the teacher labelling many of the items found in the classroom:- 'table', 'chair','window', 'book-case', 'door'. Notices are also displayed: OPEN, CLOSED, DANGER, and many other ideas can be used, e.g. the construction of an Experience Chart. Phrases and sentences may also be put up around the classroom walls – but not too many at any one time. The days of the week, the words used to describe the weather, the names of the children in the class are quite common collections used. The key words which every child needs to learn are given below (Figure 5.3).

Work with words is also carried out by children having available to them an amount of letters of the alphabet and also a stock of common words. The letters can be written on small cards or can be on small tiles (as in the game Scrabble). Alphabets consisting of the actual letters cut out from thick card or plywood are also usually available.

Many teachers make use of the system of having each child involved with three books at any one time. There is the book from which the child is learning the formal task of reading, a second book which is a story book and from which the teacher reads a story to the whole class each day, and a third book which is one the child has chosen for himself from the selection in the reading corner. This third book often goes home with the child and is used for reading to (or with) the child in the evenings. Of course, each of the three books is exchanged for another one of the same type when appropriate. Some more needs to be explained about reading schemes in case their nature and purpose is not fully appreciated.

A reading scheme is a set of books specially designed to teach reading. The vocabulary which is used in them is strictly controlled so that new words are introduced at a gradual rate, whilst the earlier words are repeated sufficiently often for them to become properly learnt. The first books of the set usually contain only a few words but are well illustrated with many attractive, colourful pictures. Increasingly often a scheme is designed which is based on research findings. Research has shown that about 100 words make up almost *half* of those in common use. In other words, very many stories can be told and ideas expressed using a comparatively small number of words out of the many thousands available to us in the English language (see Figure 5.3).

Although many children are able to learn to read from books alone, reading schemes usually have much supporting material in order to assist the teacher in her task, to provide variety in the work, and to support the slower-learning child. Hence it is quite common to find word books, wall pictures, colouring books, flash cards, tracing books, work sheets, picture dictionaries etc., all linked to a particular reading scheme being used in the classroom. Throughout, more and more words are introduced to the child and the total of words used is usually between one and two thousand.

A few other points need to be made before we move on.

Surveys have shown that *most* schools employ a *number* of reading

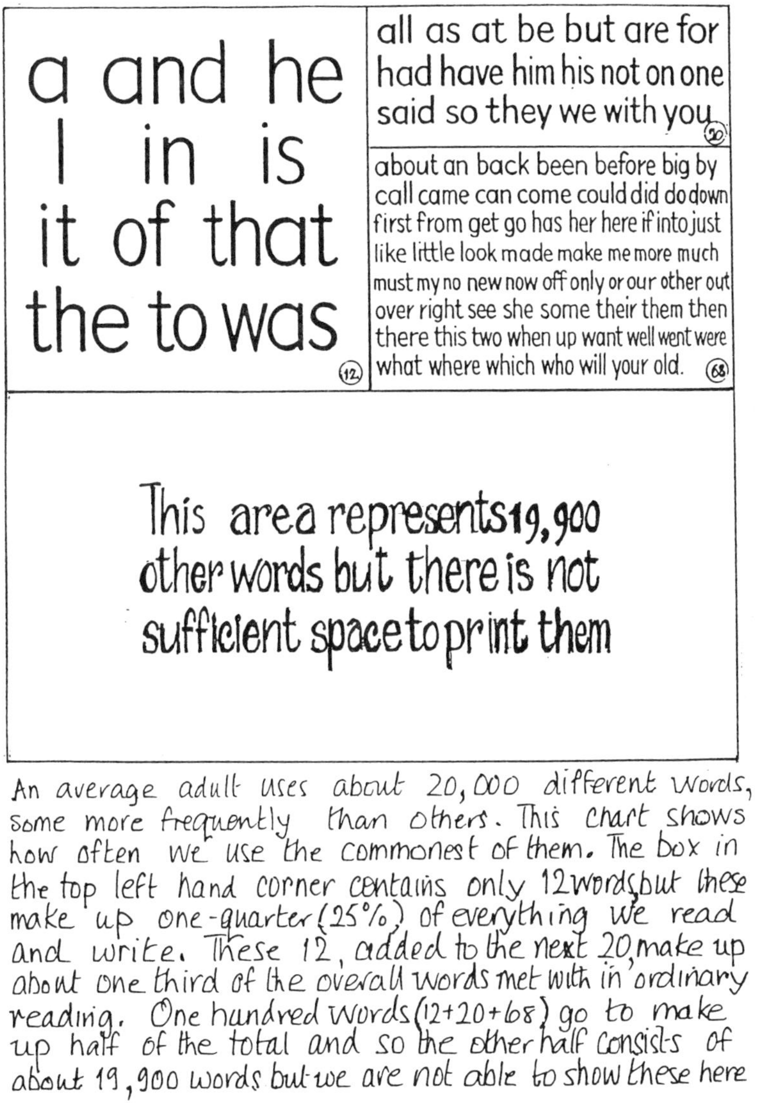

a and he

I in is

it of that

the to was (12)

all as at be but are for
had have him his not on one
said so they we with you (20)

about an back been before big by
call came can come could did do down
first from get go has her here if into just
like little look made make me more much
must my no new now off only or our other out
over right see she some their them then
there this two when up want well went were
what where which who will your old. (68)

This area represents 19,900
other words but there is not
sufficient space to print them

An average adult uses about 20,000 different words,
some more frequently than others. This chart shows
how often we use the commonest of them. The box in
the top left hand corner contains only 12 words, but these
make up one-quarter (25%) of everything we read
and write. These 12, added to the next 20, make up
about one third of the overall words met with in ordinary
reading. One hundred words (12+20+68) go to make
up half of the total and so the other half consists of
about 19,900 words but we are not able to show these here

Figure 5.3 The key words of the English language

schemes, with teachers generally being flexible in their approach
and being prepared to move from one scheme to another in order to
ensure that each child is using the most suitable book from all the
schemes available.

As has been indicated earlier, there is no clear-cut case that can be
made out in favour of either the 'look and say' or the 'phonic'

approach. Many teachers employ both approaches in their work. Typically, a teacher will start off with the 'look and say' method by building up a sight vocabulary, after which the technique of breaking down a word into the sounds of each of the component letters (or groups of letters) will be introduced. Gradually the child will build up his own skills by practice. In the case of most children both approaches are found to dove-tail together quite naturally.

In recent years – since at least 1985 – a movement has been growing with respect to the teaching of reading and which is known as the 'Apprenticeship Approach' or 'The Real Books' method. In view of its newness and ever-growing popularity we will spend some time in describing it so as, it is hoped, to provide a comprehensive overview of the whole field.

The 'Real Books' Method or 'Apprenticeship Approach' to Reading

The supporters of this method say that for the effectiveness of any approach to reading to be properly evaluated two aspects need to be considered: the QUANTITY of what is taught and the QUALITY also. (Everything in this section reflects the views of the supporters of the method).

Most schemes teach children to read quite competently in so far as children can look at a piece of writing and make out accurately what it says (the *quantity* aspect). However, many of these children fail to develop a proper love of reading (the *quality* aspect) and so read only reluctantly – often stumbling through a piece of reading almost without realising that it is supposed to make sense. It is claimed that many children exhibit no type of reaction to the books they read and apparently gain no joy at all from being able to read or from the stories in the books they have. The supporters of the 'Real Books' approach claim that the present system of teaching reading produces too many children who *can cope* with reading but who are not *readers*, as they choose to *avoid* the task of reading if at all possible.

Because of this observation it is claimed that somewhere along the line there is a failure and that the failure lies in the *approach* adopted by most teachers. It is argued that the child is best taught by treating him as if he were an apprentice to a craftsman. The teacher and child should get together (as a craftsman would with an apprentice) and be closely involved with books and all that is associated with them (in a similar manner to tools and 'tricks of the trade'). It is held that reading and writing will best be acquired in the same way that the child acquired spoken language. A child learns to talk by being surrounded by speech which the child becomes familiar with, pays attention to, works out the meaning of, and eventually starts to use etc. The child learns to speak in an environment where there is nobody making any special effort to teach him. For these reasons it is believed that it is unnatural to teach reading in any formal manner, that it is quite unnatural to introduce words in a set, regulated and controlled sequence and that effort should be concentrated *not* on getting a series of small skills to be used in a fluent manner but rather on *obtaining meaning* from the printed word.

Another belief firmly held by the supporters of the 'Apprentice-ship Approach' is that the *type of book* offered to the child to read is vitally important and that the teacher, parent or other adult is to act as a *guiding friend* to the child rather than to engage in any 'teaching' (in the generally accepted sense of the word). Books are regarded as falling into two categories: *organic* and *inorganic*.

Organic books are the only ones worth using with a child as they relate to a child's own emotions, needs and interests. They are written with the sole object in mind of telling a story and conveying a certain message or meaning. They are what children will naturally and automatically be attracted to and from which they will best learn to read. These books will sound well when read aloud. In short, they are *REAL BOOKS*.

Inorganic books, by contrast, are imposed on the child from outside and so are meaningless to him, holding, as they do, little attraction for him. Books *designed to teach reading formally* fall into this category and sound very artificial, containing, as they do, phrases and sentences that real people never say in real-life situations. These inorganic books do not, therefore, encourage any proper love of, or even regard for, reading and are to be discouraged. An example from one of these inorganic – and hence 'unreal' – books is as follows:

Go Tim
Go up
Go up Tim
Go up, up, up

The writer is attempting to make the child familiar with two short words and one short proper name by presenting them to the child repeatedly but in so doing ends up by producing a rather artificial style of language which is unlikely to be met in real life. Also, it does not read aloud well. Compare this with the first few sentences from a 'real' book:

Mr Bear was tired,
Mrs Bear was tired,
and
Baby Bear was tired,
so they all went to bed.
Mrs Bear fell asleep
Mr Bear didn't.

This writer has produced something interesting, which 'flows' well and which sounds attractive when read aloud. It is far more natural in the language that has been used and will probably be quite easy in catching the child's attention and imagination. Any teacher using the Apprenticeship/Real Books approach will make sure that the child has a wide choice of 'real' books and will help him choose one. The teacher will then read with him and generally help him become familiar with the story in the book. As time progresses the child will be able to read more and more of each book by himself, getting to know where various words and sentences occur on the page, feeling and saying the right parts of the story or rhyme etc. In short the child is invited to behave as a reader. During the process the teacher will act to ensure that the child is never made to feel a failure nor to think that there is any element of competition in what is happening.

It is not the purpose of this chapter to take sides in the long-running 'look and say' versus 'phonic' issue, or to enter into the debate that is taking place as to whether it is better to abandon both of these in favour of the 'Real Books' approach. This chapter is intended to describe what children need to learn in the process of becoming literate and to describe also some of the many skills that need to be acquired by the child when learning to read. In addition the chapter hopes to convey some idea (however rough and ready) of the methods teachers use in order to establish first the proper pre-reading skills and then to get the children started on the actual process of reading itself. The intention is also to get over the message that there is not just one particular approach to reading that is successful, and that the teaching of reading is a constantly changing process with new ideas and approaches constantly being introduced and evaluated, after which they are either incorporated into what is already ongoing or are discarded.

Before the end of the chapter it is worth making a couple of points in order to restore the proper balance to its content. In the first place we must never lose sight of the fact that the teaching of reading is very much a success story, in so far as most children leave school having achieved a satisfactory standard of literacy. Most teachers manage to teach reading quite successfully to most of the children they encounter. This holds true across a whole range of factors and is not related to any particular method(s) of teaching, or to whether the children come from high or low income groups, or to whether their schools are located in the inner cities, leafy suburbs or rural areas.

Although some people leave school illiterate or with poor literacy skills these tend to be very much in a minority. They are a cause for concern and a proportion of them are the subject of this book because of the special nature of their difficulties. But overall the teaching of reading is, and for many generations has been, largely a success story.

A second point to be made is that for the average child to learn to read adequately takes about four years to achieve. A child unable to read is considered by those involved in education to have a reading age of 5;0 years because in theory no child starts to learn to read until they go to school and 5 years is the legal starting age. Likewise, a child is considered to have reached an acceptable level of literacy if he has attained a reading age of 9;0 years. This is the reading age of an *average* child aged nine. Once a reading age of 9;0 years is attained then it is considered that the child has mastered all of the reading skills required for independent reading and that he can function adequately in society as regards reading requirements.

As time progresses it is expected that these children (with a reading age of 9;0 years) will continue to read and will progress through stories and other types of writing that contain ever more demanding vocabulary levels, i.e. longer, less common and more specialised words as well as more technical expressions etc. In short, it is expected that once a child has learned the basic skill of reading that he will then go on to become ever more proficient by using this basic skill to his maximum potential. An average child of sixteen should have a reading age of sixteen, but the increase in reading age from about nine to sixteen will be a product of *greater experience* acquired during that seven years, and not a continuation of the learning process. For them the basic rules of reading have been absorbed and the mechanisms of reading have been well practised. These pupils do not need to be given any further TEACHING as such as there are no new reading skills for them to learn. However, they need to continue with PRACTICE in their reading by moving through ever more demanding texts.

What needs to be borne in mind is that reading is a skill which is not usually acquired quickly or easily. It is a gradual process and a lengthy one. Children learn to talk and to walk in far less time than they take to learn to read. They can learn to ride a bicycle, to swim, to ice skate, to roller skate and to do so many other things in life far faster than they can become literate. The process is a complex one with no short cuts available nor any 'magic wands' that can be waved to improve matters. Learning to read requires hard work, concentration and dedication on the part of most children and these efforts need to be kept up for a considerable period of time. Even when a child is highly motivated to learn and is prepared to rise to the challenge the effort required is still quite considerable.

A dyslexic child does not respond in the way that most children do to the teaching of reading. Our next chapter looks at dyslexia itself and the one following looks at the dyslexic child in an attempt to uncover where the difficulty might lie.

Chapter 6:
Dyslexia Examined

We need to start by explaining the meaning of the word 'dyslexia' itself. The actual word 'dyslexia' has been produced from a combination of two Greek words 'dys' and 'lexicos', (the second of which has become slightly changed in the process):

'dys' means difficult, painful or abnormal;
'lexicos' means the words of a language.

Hence, dyslexia means, literally, 'a *difficulty* with *words*' and is understood to refer to written words (reading, writing and spelling) as opposed to spoken words.

As can be appreciated from this, dyslexia is merely a DESCRIPTION of a child's difficulties and can in no way be taken as an EXPLANATION of what those difficulties are or indeed anything else about them. (It may be stating the obvious, but this is the cause of at least *some* of the misunderstanding and confusion about the subject). Therefore it is illogical for a person to say, for instance, 'My child cannot read because he is dyslexic' as this is no more than saying 'My child cannot read because he has difficulty making out words written down'. It tells us no more than saying a person is bleeding badly because he has a haemhorrage or that someone has a high temperature because they are feverish. Of course a parent might say at any time, 'My child cannot read properly, because he has dyslexia' and by doing so only intends to convey the message that the poor reading is not due to the child being generally slow, or lazy or not having attended school.

Not only is the word 'dyslexia' capable of being misunderstood by people but it appears in a large number of terms ('acquired dyslexia' and 'surface dyslexia' being just two taken completely at random from a long list) as well as in association with other terms which do not contain either the word 'dyslexia' or the word 'dyslexic' but nevertheless are considered by many people to mean the same thing. ('Specific learning difficulties' and 'specific reading retardation' are two examples of this.)

Below I have listed 37 terms used in a number of books and articles about dyslexia which I surveyed for the purpose of producing this chapter. All of them are, or have been, used to refer to dyslexia at different times and by different people – doctors, psychologists, researchers etc. An explanation and/or a definition of each will be given later in this chapter.

Terms used in Relation to Dyslexia

1. acquired dyslexia
2. acute dyslexia
3. alexia
4. attentional dyslexia
5. auditory dyslexia
6. congenital dyslexia
7. congenital word blindness
8. deep dyslexia
9. developmental aphasia
10. developmental dyslexia
11. direct dyslexia
12. dyseidetic dyslexia
13. dyslexia
14. dysphonetic dyslexia
15. graphemic processor dyslexia
16. hyperlexia
17. legasthenia
18. 'L'-type dyslexia
19. mind blindness
20. mixed dyslexia
21. morphemic dyslexia
22. phonological dyslexia
23. phonological processor dyslexia
24. 'P'-type dyslexia
25. semantic processor dyslexia
26. specific developmental dyslexia
27. specific dyslexia
28. specific learning difficulties

29. specific reading difficulties
30. specific reading disabilities
31. specific reading retardation
32. strephosymbolia
33. surface dyslexia
34. traumatic dyslexia
35. visual dyslexia
36. visual processor dyslexia
37. word blindness

As can be appreciated, such a long list (and there is no guarantee that it is complete) leads to a great deal of confusion and misunderstanding. As a result a maze has grown up, through which only a comparatively small number of people can find the pathway. The majority of people become lost when they become acquainted with the subject of dyslexia for the first time. As far as many people are concerned it is by no means clear as to *why* there are so many terms, nor whether similar-sounding terms mean the same as one another. Could they refer to different but related conditions? The confusion increases when an interested parent attempts to read up about the subject and comes to learn that the use and meaning of many of the terms are challenged by some workers in the field of dyslexia. We will now attempt to find some kind of pathway through it all and, it is hoped, clear up some of the confusion.

The large number of terms associated with dyslexia is best explained to begin with by relating them to the whole range of learning difficulties that are found within the general school population. We need to start with the total population of school children and sift through them stage by stage in a gradual process of elimination until we end up with those who have dyslexia.

When the total school population is considered, it is agreed by most education workers and researchers that 80% of schoolchildren go through their school careers without any difficulty. Obviously those with dyslexia will not be found within this large, problem-free group and so we must consider the other 20%. This smaller group of 20% will experience *learning difficulties* of some sort or another at one time or another during their school lives. It needs to be explained here that the term 'learning difficulties' as used *in this context* has a very general meaning and is not to be taken in the literal sense. Because of this, children with physical handicaps or sensory difficulties are described as having learning difficulties, as are those children in delicate health or with emotional/behavioural difficulties. Any individual child who experiences these difficulties could be quite competent at general learning and be very able at reading, writing, spelling and number work. The official definition of 'learning difficulties' in the way the term is used here was set out in the 1981 Education Act and refers to *ANY* difficulty of such a nature that the child requires something *more than*, or *different from* the majority of other children of the same age in order to benefit from the education process.

Although this group of children – the 20% – need extra resources in order to benefit fully from the education process many of them do not have any difficulty with the actual process of learning itself. In fact many of them are high achievers at school.

This 20% of all children will therefore be composed of a mixture of competent readers and poor readers but the exact proportions of each are not known. Of this mixture the competent readers do not concern us and we concentrate on the remainder.

Considering the poor readers, a proportion of these will be of below-average intelligence and so their reading difficulties will be explainable by this fact. (There may be some within this group who *also* have dyslexic difficulties but these difficulties could well be masked by their general learning difficulties and might therefore be more difficult to identify.) Hence we must consider the others whose difficulties are more easily recognisable.

The remaining group – poor readers of reasonable or good intelligence – are those in whom we are interested and to whom many descriptive terms have been given. The system of identification we have just described is summarised in the flow chart in Figure 6.1. Of the 37 words on the list 10 have been mentioned in the flow chart, and it can be seen how they relate to one another. Further explanation is required to show the manner in which many of the remainder are used and how they interrelate also.

The word 'dyslexia' is, strictly speaking, a general term and refers to two distinct types:

(i)   *acquired dyslexia* – which is sometimes called *alexia*;
(ii)   *developmental dyslexia* – which is the type with which we are concerned with in this book, as it applies to children and is sometimes referred to as congenital dyslexia and at other times as specific developmental dyslexia.
        Each type will now be further explained.

Acquired dyslexia

This is sometimes called 'alexia' and also 'traumatic dyslexia' and was

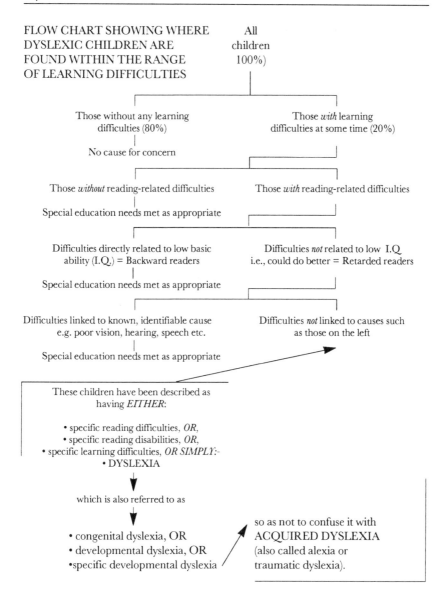

FLOW CHART SHOWING WHERE DYSLEXIC CHILDREN ARE FOUND WITHIN THE RANGE OF LEARNING DIFFICULTIES

All children 100%)

Those without any learning difficulties (80%)

No cause for concern

Those *with* learning difficulties at some time (20%)

Those *without* reading-related difficulties

Special education needs met as appropriate

Those *with* reading-related difficulties

Difficulties directly related to low basic ability (I.Q.) = Backward readers

Special education needs met as appropriate

Difficulties *not* related to low I.Q i.e., could do better = Retarded readers

Difficulties linked to known, identifiable cause e.g. poor vision, hearing, speech etc.

Special education needs met as appropriate

Difficulties *not* linked to causes such as those on the left

These children have been described as having *EITHER*:

• specific reading difficulties, *OR,*
• specific reading disabilities, *OR,*
• specific learning difficulties, *OR SIMPLY:-*
    • DYSLEXIA

which is also referred to as

• congenital dyslexia, OR
• developmental dyslexia, OR
•specific developmental dyslexia

so as not to confuse it with
ACQUIRED DYSLEXIA
(also called alexia or
traumatic dyslexia).

Figure 6.1

first identified more than a century ago. It is a condition found in medical patients (usually ADULTS) and refers to the *loss* of the ability to read which had previously been fully developed. This acquired condition results from some form of brain damage and is usually caused by accidents, tumours, strokes, drugs, psychiatric disorders or ageing. As well as being called 'alexia' the term 'word-blindness' has been used to described the same condition, all of which adds to the confusion.

In all cases of acquired dyslexia there are both 'hard' signs and 'soft' signs of brain damage. 'Hard' signs are the physical injury or wound and 'soft' signs are such features as coordination difficulties, abnormal reflexes or an unusual electroencephalogram (EEG) pattern.

Attempts were made in the mid-1970s to distinguish different syndromes of acquired dyslexia, the patients being classified into groups according to the types of reading or spelling errors that they made or the particular literacy skills that appeared to be lacking.

A survey of just five books produced in recent years (1983–91) by a total of ten editors/writers/researchers shows that six different names have been used by a variety of workers to describe sub-types of acquired dyslexia. Any particular researcher has usually claimed the existence of only two or three types and the question arises as to how close any sub-type claimed by one worker is to that claimed by another even though different names are used.

At the time of publishing their respective books the authors concerned held the posts as given below:
Colin TYRE was responsible for the Educational Psychology Service of South Glamorgan; Peter YOUNG was an editor for the Open University Press; Peter BRYANT was Watts Professor of Psychology at the University of Oxford; Lynnette BRADLEY was Senior Research Officer in the Department of Psychology at the University of Oxford; Vera QUIN and Alan MACAUSLAN ran the Learning Disabilities Clinic at St Thomas's Hospital, London; Tim MILES was Professor Emeritus of Psychology at the University College of North Wales in Bangor; Elaine MILES was Course Advisor on Teacher Training at the Dyslexia Unit of the University College of North Wales in Bangor; Peter PUMFREY was Professor of Education at the Centre for Educational Guidance and Special Needs, School of Education, Manchester University; Rea REASON was Senior Educational Psychologist at the same Centre.
The six sub-types of acquired dyslexia which are mentioned in the five books when taken together are: (1) surface (2) deep (3) phonological (4) direct (5) visual (6) attentional. The sub-types mentioned by each pair of writers is set out in Table 6.1.

As can be seen, the sub-types of surface dyslexia and deep dyslexia are mentioned in all five books, with the other three being mentioned less frequently. It is fair to say, then, that among researchers it is popularly believed that adults with acquired dyslexia do not all present as entirely the same but can be divided into sub-types. There would appear to be at least two of these but the exact

Table 6.1: Six sub-types of acquired dyslexia

		Surface	Deep	Phonological	Direct (hyperlexia)	Visual	Attentional
Young & Tyre	(1983)	✓	✓	•	•	•	•
Bryant & Bradley	(1985)	✓	✓	✓	•	•	•
Quin & Macausland	(1986)	✓	✓	•	•	•	•
Miles & Miles	(1990)	✓	✓	✓	✓	✓	✓
Pumfrey & Reason	(1991)	✓	✓	✓	✓	•	•
Total		5	5	3	2	1	1

Note ✓ = mentioned by writer(s)/researcher(s)

number is not agreed on. However, it appears more likely that there is a small number (such as two) than a large number (such as ten).

Surface dyslexics are described as reading silently 'by ear' recognising words by sounds and not by their written appearance. There is nothing wrong with their phonological skills (which will be discussed later) and they are able to read nonsense words. However, they are likely to be caught out by homophones (similar sounding words, e.g. sail/sale; where/wear; hole/whole). Often they attempt to read these words phonologically and turn them into nonsense words in doing so (e.g. *broad* read as *brode*). They have difficulty in remembering what words look like and depend heavily on working out their meaning via the rules about letter–sound relationships. Therefore their greatest difficulty is with words which cannot be read simply by letter–sound correspondence.

Deep dyslexics are described as being unable to use phonics as they are unable to connect what they see on the page with the *sound* of the word. Deep dyslexics look at a word and are likely to read it as an entirely different one, but with a related meaning (e.g. *'city'* could be read as 'Liverpool', *rose* read as *daffodil, pixie* read as *gnome*). Also, two words of similar 'shape' can be confused (e.g. *lip* can be read as *hay* as each occupies a shape like

and *punt* can be read as *gash* as the shape of each of these two is

Words which are concrete in meaning (such as man/house/tree) are more likely to be read correctly than are abstract words (such as hope/love/peace). Deep dyslexics cannot read nonsense words (e.g. nate/toge/borm) and deep dyslexia itself is considered to be the most serious sub-type of acquired dyslexia as the symptoms suggest that several components of the reading system are damaged.

Phonological dyslexia is described as being a similar, but less drastic form of deep dyslexia, involving as it does difficulties with the analysis of sounds as well as the inability to read irregular words or nonsense words. Phonological dyslexics rely heavily on the visual appearance of a word and tend to make derivational errors e.g. *weigh* can be read as *weight, wise* read as *wisdom, camp* read as *cape*). A phonological dyslexic cannot analyse a word into its phonological segments and has a tendency to add to, remove from, or change the beginning or end of a word (e.g. *thinking* can be read as *think*).

Phonological dyslexia has been described as the 'mirror image' of surface dyslexia and is a relatively recent addition to the list of sub-types of acquired dyslexia.

Direct dyslexia is often called hyperlexia. Those adults affected are accurate as regards the actual oral skills of reading but show poor comprehension of what they have read.

No information about the other claimed sub-types needs to be given here as the acquired form of dyslexia is not the main concern of this book. What has been written so far about acquired dyslexia has been solely for the purpose of rounding out the picture so that developmental dyslexia (which is the main object of our interest) can be viewed in its correct perspective, and we move on to consider it now.

Developmental dyslexia

This is the subject of this book, as it is this form of the two main types which is found in children. As seen in Figure 6.1 it is referred to by a variety of names which tends to produce some confusion. Attempts have been made by various researchers to distinguish sub-types of developmental dyslexia as it is vital to know whether all children are identical in their dyslexic reading difficulties or display two, three or even more sub-types. If all children display the same difficulties then the task facing teachers is obviously much easier as *one* teaching approach (or set of techniques) can be applied to *all* children equally.

The ten editors/writers/researchers whose work we referred to earlier describe a number of different attempts to describe sub-types of developmental dyslexia. A few brief comments will be made about each of five different classifications. There are others but these are the ones that appear to be referred to most often:

> *The Johnson and Mykelbust classification* (made in 1967) is divided into two sub-types: VISUAL dyslexics and AUDITORY dyslexics.
>
> *The Boder classification* (made in 1973) is into three sub-types: DYSPHONETIC dyslexics, DYSEIDETIC dyslexics and MIXED dyslexics.
>
> *The Seymour classification* (made in 1986) is also into three sub-types: SEMANTIC PROCESSOR dyslexics, PHONOLOGICAL PROCESSOR dyslexics and VISUAL (GRAPHEMIC) PROCESSOR dyslexics

Another researcher (Snowling) has claimed to have identified two types of children making reading errors.

> *The Snowling classification* (made in 1987) is into two sub-types: PHONOLOGICAL dyslexics and SURFACE (or MORPHEMIC) dyslexics
>
> A fifth researcher *(Bakker)* has divided developmental dyslexics into two types which he calls 'P' and 'L'. (These were proposed by him in 1990.)

These five attempts to classify developmental dyslexics are not the only attempts that have been made and each one attracts its critics. It will be noticed that three descriptions are used to describe *both* a possible type of acquired dyslexia *and* a possible type of developmental dyslexia also (surface, phonological, and visual). It must *not* be assumed that when any one of these is used in relation to acquired dyslexia that it has the same meaning when used in relation to the developmental type. We are able to summarise what we have said so far in Figure 6.2.

There is no point in describing any of the sub-types of acquired and developmental dyslexia in this chapter as they will be dealt with more fully later in the book. However, it is important for parents to realise that they feature in the research being carried out into the causes and nature of dyslexia as well as in relation to any possible means of assisting dyslexic children.

If indeed dyslexic children can be divided into sub-types then this could be an important signpost as to the cause of their condition.

DYSLEXIA

This is a general term and is used to describe TWO different conditions:

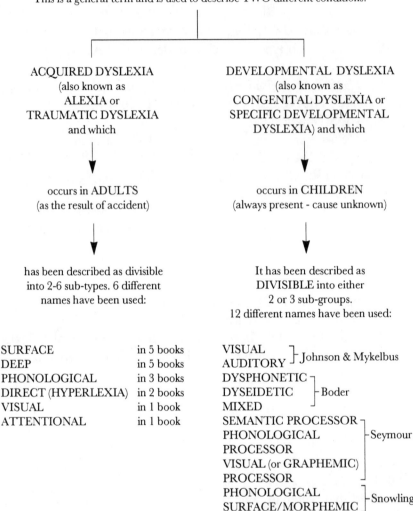

ACQUIRED DYSLEXIA
(also known as
ALEXIA or
TRAUMATIC DYSLEXIA
and which

occurs in ADULTS
(as the result of accident)

has been described as divisible
into 2-6 sub-types. 6 different
names have been used:

DEVELOPMENTAL DYSLEXIA
(also known as
CONGENITAL DYSLEXIA or
SPECIFIC DEVELOPMENTAL
DYSLEXIA) and which

occurs in CHILDREN
(always present - cause unknown)

It has been described as
DIVISIBLE into either
2 or 3 sub-groups.
12 different names have been used:

SURFACE	in 5 books	
DEEP	in 5 books	
PHONOLOGICAL	in 3 books	
DIRECT (HYPERLEXIA)	in 2 books	
VISUAL	in 1 book	
ATTENTIONAL	in 1 book	

VISUAL ⎫
AUDITORY ⎭ Johnson & Mykelbus

DYSPHONETIC ⎫
DYSEIDETIC ⎬ Boder
MIXED ⎭

SEMANTIC PROCESSOR ⎫
PHONOLOGICAL ⎪ Seymour
PROCESSOR ⎬
VISUAL (or GRAPHEMIC) ⎪
PROCESSOR ⎭

PHONOLOGICAL ⎫ Snowling
SURFACE/MORPHEMIC ⎭

'P' TYPE ⎫ Bakker
'L' TYPE ⎭

(3 sub-type names are common to both:- VISUAL, PHONOLOGICAL and
SURFACE. It must not be assumed that any of these words mean the same in both
adults and children.)

Figure 6.2 Features of acquired and developmental dyslexia

Also, if any sub-types of acquired dyslexia in adults can be found to have similarities with a sub-type of the developmental dyslexia found in children this could be a vital step to unravelling the many threads still surrounding the causes of dyslexia. A simple set of comparisons might be useful for future reference and one is set out in Table 6.2.

Table 6.2: Comparison of acquired and developmental dyslexia

Acquired type	Developmental type
• Occurs in adults	• Occurs in children
• The adults have previously learned to read	• The children have not previously learned to read
• Is a difficulty in re-establishing an already learned skill	• Is a difficulty in learning a skill
• Caused by damage to brain	Cause not known
• 'Hard' signs present in all cases	• No 'hard' signs present (in the majority of cases)
• 'Soft' signs present in all cases	• No 'soft' signs present (in the majority of cases)
• At least 6 different sub-types have been claimed	• At least 12 different sub-types have been claimed

From what we have covered so far we have learned that:

•   'dyslexia' is a word which only *describes* what a particular difficulty is, IT DOES NOT EXPLAIN ANYTHING;
•   dyslexia is a general term which covers two main types: acquired and developmental;
•   the developmental form is the type found in children;
•   both types have been called by more than one name;
•   claims have been made that each type exists in a number of different forms.

However, we have not yet attempted to explain much about dyslexia or to answer the simple but all important question: *'what is dyslexia?'* Unfortunately, there is no simple, quick or exact answer to that question, as we shall see.

When you are trying to learn something about a specialised subject with which you are not very familiar it is often a good idea to consult the experts by looking up what they have to say on the matter, and this is what has been done for the purposes of writing this chapter. Over a 21-year period, from 1968 to 1989, seven different bodies or groups of people have produced a definition of dyslexia or dyslexic-type difficulties. All of these bodies are renowned and highly respected so we can have confidence in the quality of what they have to say.

In this chapter the actual definitions themselves are *not* given here but may be found by the interested reader in the Appendix. Instead each definition has been *analysed into its component parts* and Table 6.3 has collected them together so that an easy comparison may be made.

There are five types of information displayed in the table, and these have been arranged in columns numbered 1 to 5 which we shall deal with in turn, scanning across the table from left to right.

In *Column 1* are letters A to G, each representing the SOURCE of one of the definitions concerned.

> Definition A was produced by THE WORLD FEDERATION OF NEUROLOGY in 1968;
> Definition B was produced by THE BRITISH DYSLEXIA ASSOCIATION in 1989;
> Definition C was produced by THE WORLD FEDERATION OF NEUROLOGY in 1968;
> Definition D was produced by RUTTER, TIZARD AND WHITMORE in 1970;
> Definition E was produced by TANSLEY AND PANCK-HURST in 1981;
> Definition F was produced by THE DYSLEXIA INSTITUTE in 1989;
> Definition G was produced by THE DEPARTMENT OF EDUCATION AND SCIENCE in 1972.

Column 2 tells us the NAMES used in the definitions for the reading problem(s) they are attempting to describe. Two call it *dyslexia* and two *specific learning difficulties*, others using *specific developmental dyslexia*, *specific reading retardation* or *specific reading difficulties*.

Column 3 lists the one- or two-word DESCRIPTIONS of the reading problem. Five different names are used in Column 2 and in Column 3 the reading problem is given various descriptions, two calling it a *disorder*, two using the word *problems(s)* and others *difficulty*, *low attainment* and *deficiencies*.

Column 4 sets out all the areas which are claimed to be affected (or possibly affected) by these types of reading problems. Ten different areas of the child's functioning are mentioned between the seven

Table 6.3: Seven important definitions of dyslexia/dyslexic-type difficulties

Column 1 — Origin of definition (A–G)

Column 2 — Name Used / Column 3 — How described:

	2 Name Used	3 How described
A	Dyslexia	disorder
B	Dyslexia	difficulty
C	Spec Developmental Dyslexia	disorder
D	Spec Reading Retardation	low attainment
E	Spec Learning Difficulties	problem
F	Spec Learning Difficulties	deficiencies
G	Spec Reading Difficulties	problems

4 Areas definitely/possibly affected & 5 Conditions applying:

	A	B	C	D	E	F	G	Points of agreement (out of max 7)
4 Areas definitely/possibly affected								
Reading	✓	✓	✓	✓	✓	✓	✓	7
Writing/Essay Work	✓	✓	●	●	✓	✓	✓	5
Spelling	✓	✓	●	●	✓	✓	✓	5
Number Work/Maths	●	✓	●	●	✓	✓	✓	4
General Language/Information Processing	●	✓	●	●	●	✓	●	2
Musical Notation	●	✓	●	●	●	●	✓	2
Oral Work/Speech	●	✓	●	●	●	✓	●	2
Motor Skills	●	●	●	●	●	✓	●	1
Working Memory	●	●	●	●	●	✓	●	1
Behaviour	●	●	●	●	●	✓	●	1
5 Conditions applying								
Below IQ/Ability Level	✓	●	✓	✓	●	●	✓	4
Had Been Taught	✓	●	✓	●	✓	●	●	3
Constitutional in Origin	●	✓	✓	●	●	●	●	2
Socio-cultural Opportunity	●	●	✓	●	●	●	●	1
Cognitive Disability	●	●	✓	●	●	●	●	1
Age Factor	●	●	●	✓	●	●	●	1
No Sensory Defect	●	●	●	●	✓	●	●	1
No Organic Damage	●	●	●	●	✓	●	●	1

definitions. As will be noted, *THE ONLY POINT OF AGREEMENT BETWEEN ALL SEVEN IS THAT THERE IS A DIFFICULTY WITH READING INVOLVED.* There is a large measure of agreement (5 out of 7) that WRITING and SPELLING are also involved and some agreement also (4 out of 7) that NUMBER WORK is related to the problem. After that there is very little agreement.

Column 5 details the CONDITIONS that are felt to need to apply before a child can be considered to have the type of reading difficulty with which we are concerned. In this area there is less agreement than in the factors discussed in Column 4. Only four of the definitions make a point about the child being found to perform below the standard to be expected, bearing in mind his IQ or level of basic ability. There is even less in respect of the other conditions.

It is for this reason that no easy answer can be given to the question 'What is dyslexia?' All we can say in response is that all experts agree that it is A DIFFICULTY WITH READING and that most also claim that spelling, writing and number work are affected, with peformance in these areas being below the child's basic ability level.

The fact that no exact definition has yet been produced is of little consequence. Children without reading problems learn to read in different ways and have different reading styles. Hence there is no justification in expecting that when difficulties arise they will be uniform in nature between one child and another. None of this can alter the fact that apart from those children who are poor readers because of being slow learners, THERE IS ANOTHER QUITE DISTINCT GROUP who have difficulty with reading yet are very able in other ways. These children all require early identification, adequate assessment, a proper description of their special educational needs and an appropriate level and type of specialist provision to assist them. For convenience we refer to them throughout this book as being DYSLEXIC or having DYSLEXIA. Parents, teachers and others understand these words and find them to be an easy form of verbal shorthand to describe the children with whom we are concerned.

Having dealt with dyslexia itself it is now necessary to consider the effects of dyslexia on an individual child. The dyslexic child is, therefore, the subject of the chapter which follows and should assist in rounding out the full picture of the problem.

Chapter 7:
The Dyslexic Child

The previous chapter outlined the attempts made to describe dyslexia, the different forms in which it may exist and the difficulties encountered in an attempt to define it exactly. Little was said, however, of what an actual dyslexic child is like. As dyslexia and the dyslexic child between them are the two sides of the same coin we will now fill out the other half of the picture, so to speak, by discussing the dyslexic child.

This book concentrates on dealing with the difficulties dyslexic children experience in *learning to read*. There is not the scope in a book of this nature to attempt to cover all aspects of dyslexia in depth – the others can be dealt with only briefly. Therefore reading will be given most of our attention. We know from the previous chapter that reading was the *only* area of the ten mentioned that all seven bodies agreed on. It is also the aspect of children's learning difficulties which causes most concern and on which most research has been undertaken.

However, the very fact that nine *other* areas of functioning were listed in the seven definitions is an indication of the wide variety of possible difficulties that dyslexic children can present *apart* from difficulty with reading pure and simple. As we shall learn in this chapter, there are many other causes for concern besides these nine.

The main point of this chapter can be very well illustrated if we consider as an example the case of just one child with whom I have had professional involvement. Peter was referred to the (then) Schools Psychological Service – since renamed the Educational Psychology Service – by his head teacher for assessment and advice. Figure 7.1 gives the details provided on the standard referral form. Apart from details withheld to prevent Peter, his school and the LEA being identified, the referral form is copied in full.

SCHOOLS PSYCHOLOGICAL SERVICE
Telephone:

FOR OFFICE USE ONLY   ALLOCATION

N/R

1   2
Date   Date

REFERRAL TO AN EDUCATIONAL PSYCHOLOGIST
IN ACCORDANCE WITH THE AUTHORITY'S GUIDELINES, PARENTAL AGREE-
MENT MUST HAVE BEEN OBTAINED BEFORE MAKING THIS REFERRAL

NAME: *Peter*   DATE OF BIRTH:
NAME OF PARENT(S) OR   SCHOOL:
NAME OF GUARDIAN(S)
ADDRESS: CLASS TEACHER:

TELEPHONE NO:

Please list your concerns about this child: *Concerns are academic.*
Very poor spelling/written work/reading. He is not making the
progress one would expect. He can tell a story orally but cannot
write it down. He responds intelligently in discussion. His parents
help with spelling each night with little benefit. He is unable to order
numbers. He cannot count on in 3's, 4's, 5's. Peter is willing to work
but is often frustrated.

When you discussed these concerns with the child and parents what was their
view?

Peter gets a lot of support at home and is becoming frustrated
that his younger brothers are doing better than he is.
Mrs [____] would like to know how best she can help him.

Please record the actions already taken to meet these concerns following your
discussions with the child's parents.

Peter has been assessed using the Aston Index to help guage
the extent of his problem.

Figure 7.1

What other source of help/advice have you sought e.g. S.B.R.T., E.W.O., S.C.M.O., E.G.O., Speech Therapist etc.,? (Please include copies of any relevent reports and in the case of a child who has learning difficulties, please enclose the S.B.R.T. report):

No other source of help has yet been sought

Which of the following areas of development do you feel deserve closer investigation:

Independence & Self Help	☐	Concentration & Attention	☐
Motor & Sensory	☐	Language & Communication	☑
Behaviour	☐	Motivation	☐
Attendance	☐	Emotion	☐

Academic Skills - Please state schemes used and where possible results of standardised tests.

Reading: *Starpol reading scheme.*
2·1 years behind chronological age using Schonnell last July

Spelling: *7·1 month . Vocabulary Score 10·5 using Aston Index*
Low scores on weekly tests.

Mathematics: *Major concern*
Cannot learn tables, unable to order numbers.

Other relevant information:

Peter is well-behaved and cared for. He participates in all classroom activities and has good home support. He has excellent listening skills and is a talented artist.
His performance is well below his apparent intelligence level.

Signed.............................   Date.............................

Figure 7.1 cont

Peter was just a few days short of his tenth birthday at the time of his referral. The referral details, when analysed, are found to tell an all-too-familiar story as far as dyslexic children are concerned. On the positive side, it is seen that Peter:

- can tell a story well;
- responds intelligently in discussion;
- is willing to work;
- behaves well;
- participates in classroom activities;
- has excellent communication skills;
- is a talented artist;
- listens well;
- has a high level of vocabulary;
- has parents who help him;
- gets support at home;
- has parents who requested help for him.

Despite all these factors being in his favour, however, the head teacher has to report that:

- achievement is less than Peter's ability would lead one to expect;
- there is poor spelling (almost 3 years below Peter's chronological age);
- written work is poor;
- reading ability is poor (2+ years below his chronological age);
- he is unable to put numbers in their correct sequence;
- there is an inability to count in 3s, 5s etc.;
- maths generally is a major concern;
- Peter is unable to learn his 'times' tables.

In short, Peter has a reasonably high level of intellectual ability as well as many other factors in his favour, such as concerned, supportive parents, a positive attitude to school and certain talents. Despite all these, he is poor academically, having difficulties with reading, spelling, writing and number work, and is unable to accomplish some tasks which most other children of his age achieve successfully. Many would consider Peter to be a 'typical dyslexic'.

Of course, the fact that many dyslexic children show a collection of difficulties – such as those mentioned in Peter's case – has been known for many years. Many studies have been made and reported on but one of the most detailed and interesting was that described by Professor T. Miles of the University of Bangor who has spent some decades dealing with and writing about dyslexic children.

In 1983 he published the findings gathered from testing carried out on 223 children, each of whom he considered to be 'clearly dyslexic'. (He had actually studied more than 300 but for his study he rejected all those about whom he felt doubt for any reason.) The subjects described in his study were for the most part school-age children (i.e. aged seven to seventeen) and a few older people (aged eighteen to twenty-three). There were 210 of the former and 13 of the latter. Apart from being able to describe the difficulties encountered in all 223 he was, in addition, able to select out 132 of them, each of whom he was able to match up with another, non-dyslexic child of the same gender, age and intellectual level. Thus Professor Miles was able to form a 'matched control' group by means of which he could make certain useful comparisons between dyslexic and non-dyslexic children. Much of this chapter will be concerned with summarising Professor Miles's findings but first we shall deal with a couple of matters of general interest: how many children are dyslexic and the connection between gender and dyslexia.

The Incidence of Dyslexia

Because it is not possible to define a dyslexic child exactly and in a manner which has universal acceptance, different groups of workers who have investigated reading and other related difficulties in children have studied slightly different populations and so have produced different estimates of how common dyslexia is. Apart from deciding whether a child is definitely dyslexic – and there are no clear-cut guidelines – there is also the matter of degree. A child who is dyslexic is capable of occupying any place on a range from quite slight to very marked.

Research has shown that dyslexia occurs in all groups of children irrespective of gender (but we will discuss this next), social groups, intellectual level, geographical area etc. It does not appear to be concentrated within any particular social group, ability level or part of the country. Of all the percentages quoted the one which appears to be most popular is that of 4% which, if accurate, would mean that more than two million people in the British Isles are affected. As dyslexia does *not* appear to be linked to intelligence then 4% of bright *and* of average *and* of slow-learning children will all be affected. A situation then exists such that the difficulty is likely to be *more readily identifiable* in the bright and average children than in those who are slow. The difficulties due to dyslexia in this third group of children are more likely to be overlooked because of the general learning difficulties they are experiencing anyway.

If we draw a graph of the range of children's IQs and include on it the graph of the 4% of the total population who are also dyslexic then the categories of difficulties show up clearly. There are six categories if we divide the whole population into three groups, i.e. low, average and high ability, as each of these three then sub-divide into those 4% of children with dyslexia and the other 96% without.

The graph is shown in Figure 7.2. It is necessary to show the lower graph – that relating to the dyslexic children – considerably magnified on the vertical scale for the purpose of clarity. This bottom graph is, therefore, drawn at a level ten times higher than it would normally be and, when looking at the graph, proper allowance must be made for this deliberate distortion.

The six groups into which the children fall have been marked on the graph. The groups are:

LW = *L*ow ability and *W*ithout dyslexia (producing single difficulty);
LD = *L*ow ability but with *D*yslexia (producing double difficulty);
AW = *A*verage ability and *W*ithout dyslexia (producing no difficulty);
AD = *A*verage ability but with *D*yslexia (producing single difficulty);
HW = *H*igh ability and *W*ithout dyslexia (producing no difficulty);
HD = *H*igh ability but with *D*yslexia (producing single difficulty).

As we can see, two groups experience no difficulty of any kind (those of average or high intelligence and without dyslexia), three groups experience a single difficulty (dyslexia in two cases and low ability in the other) and one group is unfortunate enough to have a double difficulty. This last group – the children who are of low basic ability and in addition have dyslexia – happen also to be the ones who are most difficult to diagnose because of the 'masking' effect referred to above. Furthermore, the same group of children is also likely to contain those who prove the most difficult to assist once they are identified. This situation can be summarised as in Table 7.1.

As a final word on this topic, it has been suggested by some workers that dyslexia should be considered to be present only in those children of *at least average* intelligence and that the description 'dyslexia' should not be applied to children in the low ability range.

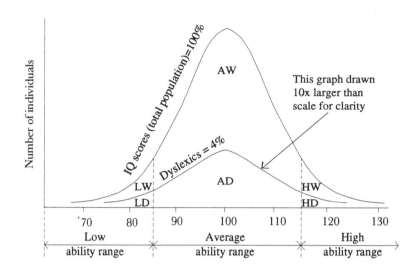

Figure 7.2

Table 7.1: The range of children's IQs and the categories of difficulties

Group	Number of difficulties	Ease of detection	Ease of remediation
LW	1	-	-
LD	2	Difficult	Difficult
AW	0	-	-
AD	1	Moderate	Moderate
HW	0	-	-
HD	1	Good	Good

Dyslexia and Gender

Although both boys and girls can have dyslexia it is a matter of fact that about four times more boys than girls are found to be dyslexic. (That is one of the reasons that throughout this book I have referred to the dyslexic child as 'he'.) As with so many other aspects of dyslexia, exact figures are difficult, if not impossible, to arrive at and some estimates have placed the proportions as high as *seven* to one but the lower figure would appear to be more likely (Professor Miles found that in the children he surveyed there were just over four to one).

We now move on to the main body of the chapter.

Professor Miles's Survey Results

Reading

In the great majority of cases where a dyslexic 'pattern' of difficulties is found then some aspect of reading difficulty will be found. In by far the majority of cases reading was affected but there are occasional cases where reading difficulty does not appear to be the major problem. Of his 232 subjects, 191(86%) could be described as poor and another 24 (11%) as fairly poor. (Unfortunately Professor Miles does not use exact measurements.) He concludes that for many dyslexics there will be difficulty in learning to read but that the skill will eventually be mastered. However, they are likely to remain slow readers and reading aloud could present particular problems for them.

Spelling

No figures are given which summarise the findings but a detailed analysis was made of the *types* of spelling error found. Dyslexic children show bizarre spellings – as do non-dyslexic children who are 'out of their depth'. Some errors are plausible in so far as words *could* be spelled that way but in fact are not (e.g. 'asist' for 'assist') whereas bizarre spellings reveal that the children concerned have little or no knowledge of the relationship that exists between letters and the sounds they represent. Professor Miles has been able to give details of 13 different types of spelling error altogether.

Left–Right Confusion

In all, 149 of the 223 children (67%) showed uncertainty over left and right. The control sample was able to be employed in this, when it was found that 87 of the 132 dyslexics (66%) showed confusion compared with only 36% of the control group. Many dyslexic children showed general uncertainty in tasks and were also confused about their body parts (right leg, left ear, right eye etc.) and the body parts of others. In attempting to give directions to people they made more errors than other children. Even a child who knew the words 'port' and 'starboard' used them incorrectly.

Many right-handed children were helped by remembering the phrase 'I *write* with my *right*'. Many, when young, need to have gloves and shoes specially marked in some way and others make use of body markings such as freckles or scars. It is also common for a dyslexic child to distinguish left from right by means of remembering on which wrist they wear their watch or on which hand they wear their ring etc. There is good reason to believe that it is only the words 'left' and 'right' which cause the difficulty, not the actual directions themselves as in many circumstances they function normally.

East–West Confusion

No statistics were given but the findings were collected mainly from the older children in the survey. Some dyslexic children are confused about direction and the degree of confusion is related to age because it is only as children get older that they learn there are four compass points to be used in describing direction and movement about the world.

Confusion over east and west appears greater than any other kind of difficulty but a detailed description of directional errors is not possible.

'b' and 'd' Confusion

In all, 146 children, or 65%, showed this type of confusion and Professor Miles felt that there was good reason to think this an underestimate as it was likely that some of the older children had experienced this difficulty when younger. This type of difficulty turned out to be particularly persistent as some children in the higher age range still experienced the confusion. Of course it is not only dyslexic children who confuse 'b' and 'd' but another study (by Bottomley) showed that three times as many errors were made by dyslexics as by non-dyslexics *who had the same spelling age* (as distinct from having the same chronological age).

The letters 'b' and 'd' were not the only letters to be confused. Mistakes over 'p' and 'q', as well as over 'p' and 'b' were reported. These confusions clear up as children get older but the 'b' and 'd' error persists longer. Professor Miles attributes this to the fact that the *sounds* of this pair of letters are so similar.

Times and Dates Confusion

No statistics were given but the fact of confusion is noted. Dyslexic children can be late in learning to tell the time and experience difficulty in remembering the days of the week in correct sequence. However, the abstract *concept* that the passage of time is marked by days of the week etc. is as well *understood* by dyslexics as by other children.

Recall of Months of the Year

In the survey 55% of the total could not recite the months of the year
in correct order. When the control group was employed it was found
that 57% of dyslexics were unsuccessful, compared with 20% of the
controls. In addition, some did not know at which month to start the
sequence. Many had to resort to memory aids. However, the months
of the year do get learned as older children did better than the
younger ones.

Subtraction and Addition

No statistics are given indicating what percentage of the dyslexic
children experience difficulties with these two basic types of calculation, but the observation is made that the difficulties fall into three
groups:

(i)   those showing a *basic* weakness related to calculation in general;
(ii) those showing a particular uncertainty in relation to the *direction*
      of the number series;
(iii) those who needed to use compensatory strategies.

The first type suggests that one cannot assume that a dyslexic child
will acquire the basic knowledge of numbers and how they behave
just as other children acquire it during the course of everyday experiences at home and school. The second type suggests that there is
particular difficulty in getting numbers the correct way round: '7
take away 5' could be confused with '5 take away 7', '62' could be
written as 26 and '38' could be read as '83'. (Uncertainty over left
and right could well be part of the reason.)

Compensatory strategies used were techniques such as counting
on fingers or making marks on paper or even drawings, depending
on the type of problem they were asked to solve. Despite needing
these, the overall picture was one of basically capable children who
were quite severely restricted in their ability to carry out some simple
mental arithmetical calculations.

Reciting Tables

The statistics showed that difficulties over tables are found not only
in dyslexic children – 89% of the total of 223 showed difficulties and
on the 'matched controls' comparison there were 90% of dyslexics
and 54% of non-dyslexics. Children tended to lose their place when

reciting, made errors of various kinds and often needed to use their fingers to assist them.

Dyslexic children are normally at an older age than others before a set of tables is eventually mastered. Professor Miles found that at age 13 years some of his subjects could still not recite the 3x and 4x tables and in fact the age of 16 years was the earliest at which these two tables no longer presented problems.

Recall of Digits

The survey contained the results of testing all 223 subjects on digits presented to them *auditorily* but the results of *visually* presented digits were available on only 42 of these as this type of test was not introduced until some time after the survey had got under way.

The 42 children concerned thereby provided the opportunity for a comparison to be made of these two sensory channels. In the case of auditorily presented digits (i.e. strings of numbers read out to the child by Professor Miles) dyslexic children could not, for the most part, remember as many numbers as others of the same age. (This was true whether they had to recite back the numbers in the order given or in reverse.)

In the case of visually presented digits the numbers were flashed up on a screen in front of the children, the numbers being made visible for an exact length of time by means of a special machine. It was possible to vary the number of digits shown at any one time and also to vary the exposure time. Dyslexic children took longer than non-dyslexics to perceive the numbers correctly. When the 42 subjects who had been tested both auditorily and visually were subjected to auditory ability–visual ability comparison it was found that they did *not* fall into the two groups and so it was *not possible* to describe some of them as 'auditory dyslexic' (having an auditory weakness but no visual weakness) and others as 'visual dyslexic' (the converse). Children who scored high on the visual condition did *not* necessarily score low on the auditory condition, and the converse also applied. It appears from this that most dyslexic persons find it difficult to process symbolic verbal material irrespective of which channel is used.

Memory for Sentences

When given a sentence and asked to repeat it back many dyslexic children could not do so word-for-word. In most cases the *sense* of what was said to them was accurately perceived and repeated back but there was difficulty in getting the actual wording correct.

Other Memory Problems

Some dyslexic children are reported to have difficulty in learning *nursery rhymes* and also *the alphabet.*

Copying from the Blackboard

This was also mentioned as a difficulty on many occasions.

Learning a Foreign Language

Difficulty with a foreign language was often reported; often a dyslexic child can be good at the oral part but have difficulty with writing the language concerned.

Finding Rhymes

Professor Miles reports that a small number of the dyslexic children found difficulty in learning a word to rhyme with another word given, e.g., 'a colour which rhymes with *head*'. 'a number which rhymes with *tree*' etc. He felt that they had somehow 'missed out' – were at a loss to know what was required. (The existence of a difficulty on the part of poor readers over recognising whether words rhyme has also been reported by two researchers: Bradley and Bryant.)

Bell-ringing

Although this may seem rather curious, two of the subjects in the survey had attempted to learn bell-ringing but had had to give it up because they could not keep count!

Driving a Car

Concerns are often expressed, usually because of confusion over 'left' and 'right', but it would appear that the confusion relates only to the words and not to the actual directions. There is no reason to think that dyslexic car drivers cannot be good drivers or that they are involved in more traffic accidents than others.

Chess

Dyslexia should not cause any difficulties in chess playing and many dyslexic children are successful at chess. No memory overload is involved as the different moves can be considered separately and do not need to be held in mind all at once.

Music

Some of the subjects in the survey were gifted musically. Any draw-back from dyslexia would relate to the *reading* of musical notation, not the basic appreciation of the music itself. However, the correct reading of written music could be learned eventually as can learning to read a book.

Art and Craft

Those talents least affected by dyslexia will be the ones most likely to flourish in dyslexic children. Art is one subject in which there are few, if any, dyslexic-type difficulties to overcome. Woodwork, pottery and other craftwork can also be produced to the highest standards.

Creative Writing

As Professor Miles puts it, 'Many of my subjects showed remarkable powers of literary appreciation and expression'. Many of the school books he saw contained lovely imaginative writing and poetry, albeit often badly spelled and with crossings-out. As he summed it up: 'A weak lexical system appears to be no barrier to creative writing'.

The overall picture presented is that a dyslexic child, apart from having difficulty in learning to read, is likely to have difficulty in a number of other areas of learning and school progress. It is not poss-ible to say which areas of the child's functioning are likely to be affected as no two children will be exactly alike and even in two with the same areas affected there are quite likely to be differences of degree between one and another.

As far as school work is concerned, reading, writing, number work (the three Rs), together with spelling, are the ones on which progress is most firmly based and so will cause the most concern if deficient. Other factors, such as confusion over left and right or an inability to put the months of the year in correct order, are likely to be viewed as irritations rather than as major difficulties and so will produce less concern. Knowing about them certainly helps to round out the overall picture presented by the child and can be an indication of how much he will need to overcome.

Up to now in this chapter we have, if anything, described the picture likely to be presented by the young child when first referred for a psychological assessment of his learning difficulties so that appropriate advice may be given. We shall now look forward and consider what lies ahead.

Professor Miles was unable to carry out a longitudinal study, much as he would have liked to do so. Most of his subjects were seen by him only once and he was unable to follow them up in the years after he had seen them. Hence he was unable to report on the progress they made. However, because his subjects embraced a wide range (most being from seven to seventeen years of age) he was able to do the next best thing and compare one age-group with another, with the results given below.

Reading Progress

The older subjects were much more successful at reading than the younger ones, the average scores on the reading test he used increasing from 18 at age seven to 92 at age eighteen. This bears out the results of many other investigations that show dyslexic children do improve over time, the rate of progress being likely to depend on how favourable the conditions are under which they are being taught.

Spelling Progress

This also improved over time. At age seven the average spelling score was 13 but it was found to be 64 in those who were ten years older. There was a steady improvement, year on year.

Four other tests were studied: digits forward (i.e. ability to remember a string of digits), digits reversed, months forward and months reversed. In these four tasks the older subjects were only slightly more competent than the younger ones.

Professor Miles was, in fact, able to do a full reassessment of 21 of his subjects at intervals which varied from as little as 7 months to as long as 7 years 7 months. Gains in reading age were recorded from 1 year 4 months to 6 years 0 months. On average each child had increased his or her reading age by 1 year for each year that had elapsed. In other words, since being assessed for the first time, their reading had 'kept up with the clock'. In the same way, spelling was found to have improved by 9 months for each year that had elapsed. Assessment would appear to have made a difference!

The general evidence from this shows that dyslexic children can improve their performance in all kinds of ways as they grow older and that, even at reading and spelling, there can be appreciable gains if the conditions are right. Even so, it is clear that traces of the handicap remain.

Now that we have a clear picture of a dyslexic child our next task is to discuss his assessment. For a child to be assisted there must first be an adequate assessment. However, the matter is not always a straightforward one and can give rise to controversy. The next chapter is intended to give a full description of the process and to clarify some of the confusions that can arise from time to time.

Chapter 8:
Assessment of the Dyslexic Child

Each year many children with reading difficulties suspected of being caused by dyslexia reach the stage where an educational psychologist is called in to carry out an assessment. When this stage is reached the assessment needs to be carried out by observing the same basic rules that should apply to any assessment of any type of difficulty in any child by any educational psychologist.

Basically, the assessment of a learning difficulty (or difficulties) in a child is an attempt to produce the answer to a question by means of investigative techniques. The question in the case of the type of child with which we are concerned in this book is usually, 'Is my child dyslexic?' or 'Does my child have a specific learning difficulty(ies)?'

The assessment should always be a sufficiently full one to produce an answer to the problem posed. More than that, it should also be full enough to be able to justify the answer given. The question could well be asked as to what is a *full* assessment, and misunderstandings sometimes arise in regard to the assessment of a child as to whether a 'full' assessment is necessary, or has been requested or has been carried out. A 'full' assessment has never been defined and is probably unlikely ever to be so. At the present time there are hundreds, if not thousands of tests, scales, screening devices, profiles, questionnaires etc. designed to gather information about children's skills, abilities, aptitudes, strengths, weaknesses, deficiencies, intelligence, perception etc., so that no matter how many are applied to a child there will always be some that have not been used. Obviously, a common-sense approach is required. Provided that the assessment of the child is full enough to answer the basic question and so address the difficulty giving rise to concern, then the assessment should be regarded as a full one. In fact it could be argued that once sufficient assessment has been carried out in order to provide a diagnosis of the difficulty and the educational psychologist is able to explain the diagnosis she has arrived at, then further assessment is not justified and could be considered a waste of scarce and costly resources (professional's time, pro formas etc.).

The educational psychologist, then, in her assessment has the general aim of investigating the child referred to her and carrying out an assessment of sufficient depth as to diagnose why the child has the difficulties described. There are many other aims, such as to be able to explain the reasons for the conclusions reached, to make recommendations as to how the child might best be assisted in his difficulties, to provide a report setting out a description of the child so that all those concerned with his education and development can be properly informed about his functioning etc.

Different local education authorities (LEAs) have different procedures to be followed when a schoolchild is referred for assessment by an educational psychologist and every educational psychologist has her (or his) own way of working. Because of this, some of what follows will vary in detail between LEAs and even within any one particular LEA. However, the general outcome should be similar.

Educational Psychologist's Interview/Assessment

In order to assess a child an educational psychologist must gather information. This comes from a number of sources, usually the school, the parents and the child himself. The information is often in written form (e.g. school records and reports) or is gained from interview(s). There is also what the psychologist learns from the child himself – by observing, by interviewing and by carrying out standardised tests.

All sources of information are important and sometimes a vital piece of information comes from a very unexpected source – often in the form of a chance remark or afterthought. During the assessment process the psychologist must gather as much information as she can.

Background Information

Basic details are all important and should not be overlooked. The spelling of the child's name needs to be checked as well as the date of birth. Sometimes these are inaccurate in the initial set of details provided, and if so could have serious implications. It is also necessary to know whether the child has ever been known by another name as hospitals and other agencies could well have records under the previous identity.

The child's educational history can say so much. Has the child attended just one school, has he been to two or have there been frequent changes? What has been the pattern of attendance – quite full, a few lengthy absences or long runs of broken weeks?

Developmental and medical history requires thorough investigation and needs to cover subjects such as eyesight, hearing, speech development, accidents, illnesses, need of period(s) as hospital in-patient. Obviously anything of significance which arises will need to be investigated in more detail and this could, in turn, lead to further lines of investigation.

Some knowledge of family background is vital – the size and structure of the family, and who presently lives in the child's home. An only child with both parents at home is living under very different conditions from another who is one of five with a single parent. The first child might be able to call on more support at home than might the second when it comes to bringing a reading book home from school and hoping to have an adult listen to him. All other aspects of family life will affect a child's development – financial circumstances, material state of the home, the general environment, interpersonal relationships etc., but the extent of the influence of each is a matter of judgement, taking all other factors into account. When investigating a child suspected of being dyslexic it is necessary to enquire also into whether there is any history of reading difficulties in the family – particularly in respect of brothers, sisters, parents, grandparents, aunts and uncles.

Up to this point the information has related only to the child's background and is of a very general nature. It could be argued that much if not all of it should be gathered in the case of every child referred to an educational psychologist, not just those suspected of being dyslexic. After the gathering of as much basic information as circumstances permit, the child himself needs to be interviewed and tested.

No two children are identical and so no two cases referred to an educational psychologist can be identical either. Therefore, there is no strictly laid-down pattern of activity which an educational psychologist must carry out in her work; it would be impossible to produce one which would apply in all cases. Most educational psychologists proceed in their work by drawing up in their mind a list of possible explanations (normally called hypotheses) as to why the child has the difficulty displayed. This mental list is arranged in descending order from the most likely down to the least likely explanation. The educational psychologist then goes on to test out the most likely one.

If it is confirmed by the test results, then well and good. If it is not confirmed then that particular hypothesis is abandoned and the next one on the list is similarly tested out. This process continues until one is – or appears to be – confirmed and matters proceed from there. (Sometimes the testing out takes place over a period of time as the psychologist recommends that a particular teaching technique be used and then time must be allowed in order for it to be properly put to the test.)

Testing

When an educational psychologist starts to assess a child referred to her as possibly dyslexic she will need to establish two basic facts as a starting point (as we have described in earlier chapters). These are

(i)   How well should the child be *expected* to read?
(ii)   How well (or badly) is the child *actually* reading?

Intelligence

As has been described in an earlier chapter, the answer to (i) depends principally on two factors – the child's age and level of intelligence. All other things being equal, a child's reading age should be equal to his chronological age. However, in many cases all other things are *not* equal and one of the greatest influences on a child's ability to read will be his intelligence level. Because of this a child of high intelligence should have a higher reading age than a child of average intelligence and of the same age. Similarly the child of average intelligence should read better than a child of low intelligence and of the same age. In other words, a child's reading age should match his mental age, as we have explained fully earlier.

The answer to (i) is thus provided by the administration of a suitable intelligence scale (or test, to use the popular name for it). I have described the WISC in detail in an earlier chapter and will also refer to it here for the sake of continuity. The educational psychologist will be interested in much more than the final IQ figure. She will need to administer 11 sub-tests (6 verbal and 5 performance) and from them will gain such information as:

(a) the overall, full-scale IQ;
(b) the verbal and performance IQs. These will need to be compared to see how closely they correlate;

(c) the individual verbal sub-test scaled scores (6 of them) in order to see the *range* displayed and the *pattern* exhibited;

(d) the individual performance sub-test scores (5 of them) for the same reason as in (c). She will then be able to arrive at some conclusion as to the level at which the child should be reading.

Reading

The answer to (ii) – At what level is the child *actually* reading? – is answered by the administration of a reading test or, what is often more informative, by a *number* of reading tests. There are a number of aspects to reading, any or all of which might repay investigation depending upon the circumstances of any individual child's case.

It can be useful to know how well a child can read single words where there is no chance of his picking up clues from what else is written when he is not quite sure of the word. It is also useful to know how well he reads individual sentences, as well as continuous prose. When a child has read a piece of print, even though he has read out each word correctly, it is useful to know just how much he has actually *understood* of what he has just read, and so a measure of the child's comprehension of print is valuable in diagnosing difficulties. Speed of reading is yet another factor as a child can read something quickly, at average speed or extremely slowly and it might be considered necessary to have a measure of this particular reading skill.

The remainder of the assessment procedure will very much depend on whether other difficulties are present, if so in what concentration, and to what degree.

Spelling

Spelling difficulties invariably accompany reading difficulties and indeed it would be unusual if this were not so. A spelling test will establish a spelling age, and examination of the types of errors the child made when attempting to spell words too difficult for him can yield useful clues to his difficulties.

Writing

Writing may also be a problem for a child with learning difficulties and can be examined from a number of viewpoints.

Ability to copy might need to be tested. Irrespective of how accurately the child is able to reproduce what is before him, the *speed* at which the copying is executed could well be a major difficulty.

Ability to take dictation could also repay investigation and be examined for spelling errors, punctuation difficulties and speed.

Free writing will produce further information about spelling, punctuation, grammar, syntax, sentence structure and ability to express ideas, as well as speed of execution.

Whilst assessing a child's writing skills – or lack of them – the type of pen grip the child employs will need to be considered, as will also whether the child is left-handed. Other factors, often given little attention, might need to be examined. These would include the manner in which the child sits on his chair, positions himself at his desk or table, has his book or sheet of paper in front of him, how he holds it steady when writing, etc.

Other Test Results

Although circumstances will differ from one particular case to another it can be said *as a generalisation* that any further testing/assessment carried out on a child considered to be dyslexic (on the basis of the results produced up to this point) will tend to provide information about accompanying problems or further insight into what type of dyslexic difficulties are involved.

It is argued by some that any assessment should look at such aspects of the child's functioning as laterality, left–right awareness, eye dominance and fine-motor control as well as commenting on matters such as short-term memory, long-term memory, visual skills (such as sequencing and perception) and auditory skills. Others take the view that whilst such items of information are useful to have, they are not necessary as they are not likely to be of overriding significance. From the pragmatic point of view a limit needs to be drawn somewhere and, providing sufficient assessment has been carried out to address the difficulties described, further assessment is desirable but probably not essential. After the basic data have been gathered there is likely to be a situation of diminishing returns arising, such that it will require ever-increasing amounts of professional man-hours of assessment to obtain progressively smaller (and probably less relevant) amounts of information about the child.

After the Assessment

For a number of good reasons the educational psychologist's assessment might need to be spread over two or more sessions. However many sessions it takes, the child's assessment will eventually be complete and a discussion of the findings will then take place between the psychologist and the parent(s).

This is obviously a valuable opportunity for the parent to compare his or her own impression of the child's difficulties with the psychologist's in order to see how closely they match. If there is a mismatch at any point then this can be talked through – it is hoped until the parent is satisfied. Any questions in the parent's mind should be put to the educational psychologist for her to answer and any points about which they would like a discussion should be brought up. Differences should also be brought out and eventually each should know what is in the mind of the other regarding the child's difficulties. The parent should ask him or herself a number of questions such as:

- Does the assessment appear to have been a reasonably full one?
- Does the description of my child's strengths and weaknesses agree with what I know?
- Have I had my questions answered?
- Have I had any areas of doubt on my part cleared up?
- Have I learned anything new?
- If I have been told anything which I was not aware of before does it appear to fit into the overall picture I have of my child?

This set of questions is not supposed to be exhaustive but rather to indicate the lines along which any parent–psychologist discussion should proceed after the assessment is completed. Eventually a report will be provided and this should be a clear and concise summary of what has been discussed. A suggested layout of a report follows:

Loamshire Educational Authority
Main Road
Newtown

22 October 1993

Educational Psychology Service

Educational Psychologist's report on:
John BROWN (dob = 6 July 1985)
26 Canal Street, NEWTOWN (N16 7BR)
Springfield JMI School

Referral details

John was referred to the Loamshire Educational Psychology Service in mid-September 1993. Both parents and school had been concerned for some time about the difficulties John exhibited in reading, spelling and writing. Despite close home/school liaison and cooperation involving extra tuition in school from a member of the LEA's support teaching team and extra reading practice at home each evening, John did not make the improvements hoped for. In other aspects of school work and life in general John was no cause for concern.

The general impression given was of a child of at least average ability overall who enjoyed school and participated fully in school activities. He was reported as being a good conversationalist, able to express his feelings well orally but finding difficulty with printed work and any work which involved writing.

John was seen by me in school on two occasions, 15 and 19 October 1993, and on the former of these I was also able to interview his parents who attended as invited. I was also able to discuss matters with his previous and present class teachers as well as read the school file relating to John.

Throughout the two sessions John was pleasant and relaxed. He cooperated well with the tasks set and in answering the questions put to him. I would report as follows:

Background details

John, who is aged 8 years 3 months, is the younger of a family of two children, there being a ten-year-old sister (Stephanie). He lives with his sister and both parents. Mr Brown is presently in full-time paid employment working regular hours and Mrs Brown is a full-time housewife and mother.

John is presently in the second year of the Junior Department of Springfield School (i.e. a National Curriculum Year 4 child). Stephanie also attends Springfield and is in Year 6. John's education commenced with his spending a year in the nursery class at Springfield, after which he enrolled in the reception class and has progressed through the school to date. With his birthday falling towards the end of the academic year he is one of the youngest children in his year group.

Mr and Mrs Brown report that there are no significant incidents or episodes to relate in John's general development. He attained his developmental milestone at or before the expected times, has experienced only the normal childhood ailments, has not had any serious accidents or illnesses and has never needed to spend a night in hospital. John has also been a regular and punctual attender at school, his record showing very few periods of absence and each of these being of relatively short duration. He has attended only the one primary school and has remained with the same peer-group throughout. The family have lived at the same address since John was two years old and have not experienced any significant disruptions to family life.

Neither Mr nor Mrs Brown experience any difficulty with reading etc. and neither has a history of any such difficulties. Stephanie does not exhibit the difficulties displayed by John and Mr and Mrs Brown are not aware of any difficulties with reading in either family background.

Functioning

John's *intellectual ability* was assessed using the WISC-R/S, and produced the following results:

Verbal Sub-tests (scaled scores)
Information   6
Similarities   17
Arithmetic   6
Vocabulary   14
Comprehension   16
(Digit Span)   (6)   (Total = 59)

Performance Sub-tests (scaled scores)

Picture Completion   12
Picture Arrangement   11
Block Design   12

Object Assembly   14
Coding   7   (Total = 56)

Verbal IQ = 110, Performance IQ = 108, Full-scale IQ = 110

As can be seen, John's verbal scores range from 6 to 14, a spread of 8 which is greater than would normally be expected, and is demonstrated by only a small proportion of the population. His performance scores are relatively tightly banded together with the exception of coding. (For a fuller explanation of the WISC scores and their significance please refer to the enclosed information sheet headed 'WISC – description'.)

John is a boy of average intelligence overall and his verbal IQ of 110 lies at the top of the range of 85–115. This score of 110 masks a pattern of underlying strengths and weaknesses which need to be considered when taking John's overall functioning into account. Such a type of pattern will be present in only a small percentage of the population.

John's *reading* ability was assessed using the Neale Analysis of Reading Ability with the following results:

Reading Age   (Rate)   = 6y 3m
Reading Age   (Accuracy)   = 6y 7m
Reading Age   (Comprehension)   = 7y 1m

As can be seen, John scores significantly below his anticipated attainment level in all three reading skills assessed. He reads at the speed of a child aged 6 years 3 months but has an accuracy level some 4 months greater than this. John's level of comprehension produces the highest score, as would be anticipated from his measured level of intelligence. In this, however, he is still attaining a level which is more than one year below his chronological age and two years below what would be anticipated, taking his basic ability into account.

John's *spelling* was assessed using the Daniels and Diack test and was found to be at the 6 years 6 months level which accords well with his reading accuracy age.

John's *writing skills* were examined under three different sets of conditions:

1. Copying This resulted in small, neat, easily-legible writing. There were errors relating to punctuation, e.g. i's not dotted, t's not crossed, full stops omitted etc. However, John's biggest difficulty was his extremely slow writing speed. It took him just over five minutes to produce a passage of fourteen words.

2. Dictation In this the style of writing remained unchanged but many spelling errors were displayed. John's writing was legible but some words could be made out only with difficulty. There was a higher percentage of punctuation errors and the writing was also executed slowly.

3. Free Writing John produced a piece of free writing. The result was almost completely illegible due to a high proportion of words misspelled. Most of these were as a result of John attempting to spell an unknown word phonetically. When John was asked to read back this short passage he was able to do so only with some difficulty and it is likely that he would not have been able to do so with a piece of work done some days earlier. However, the content of his writing was of good quality for a child of his age. Speed of writing remained a problem in this exercise also.

Recommendations

The results show that John is a child of above-average ability who displays specific difficulties of a dyslexic type in the areas of reading, spelling and writing. In my opinion he has special educational needs which, to be met, require the provision of:

1. teaching individually or in a small group;
2. the teaching to be given on a daily basis, the sessions to be of 30 minutes' duration initially and to be adjusted at intervals according to the rate of progress;
3. the teacher to have experience of teaching children with dyslexia/specific learning difficulties;
4. teaching to concentrate on improving:

    (i)   reading speed;
    (ii)   reading accuracy;
    (iii) spelling;
    (iv) general writing skills.

Signed ....

Educational Psychologist

Figure 8.1 The educational psychologist's report

(The separate information sheet referred to in the report follows).

WISC: description

The WISC (which stands for the Wechsler Intelligence Scale for Children) is the most widely used test of general intelligence designed for children and allows assessment to take place of a child's problem-solving abilities.

The Full-scale IQ summarises overall performance and provides a broad assessment of general intelligence and the ability to do well in school.

The assessment takes place along two dimensions, the *verbal* (using words) and the non-verbal (or *performance*) (by using hand and eye skills).

The Verbal IQ is generally based on performance in the first five of the six verbal sub-tests and the Performance IQ is similarly based on the first five of the six performance sub-tests. The Verbal IQ provides an indication of verbal comprehension, including the ability to use verbal skills in reasoning and solving problems as well as the capacity to learn verbal material.

The Performance IQ reflects the efficiency and integrity of the child's perceptual organisation, including non-verbal reasoning skills, the ability to employ visual images in thinking and the ability to process visual material.

The sub-test scaled scores all range from 1 to 19 with the average score for all children being 10 and most scores grouped within a range of 8 to 12.

The IQs of both Verbal and Performance Scales range from 65 to 135 with the average scores for all children being 100. The Verbal and Performance IQs of most children match one another quite closely, a discrepancy of a few points being quite common but larger discrepancies (e.g. 12 or more) being found in only about 5% of the population.

The Full-scale, Verbal and Performance IQs may be influenced by a variety of factors.

This report is only a suggested format and is not being put forward as beyond criticism. However, I do believe that it covers all the essentials in the case of the fictitious child concerned, and also provides useful guidelines to the teacher who will undertake work with John. Of course, other aspects of John's functioning could have been investigated and reported on but whether any highly relevant information would result is a matter for conjecture.

The report produced describes the difficulties John is experiencing, details the assessment carried out, the results obtained and the conclusions drawn. It goes on to specify in *general* terms how John would best be helped, the finer details of the teaching programme being left for John's special needs teacher. She will be able to decide on the approach to adopt, the design of the individual programme to be used, the pattern of work in each session, the type and amount of home practice required by John each evening, etc.

Other factors could have been mentioned – such as those relating to personality, social adjustment, emotional difficulties and behaviour. Some people would argue that they should always be investigated and reported on. My own practice is to refer to them only if such extremes are displayed as are likely to affect the teaching programme.

Parental Satisfaction

Throughout the assessment procedure there should be parental agreement with the suggestions made, the steps taken, the contents of the report and the help offered. If there is any disagreement or dispute then it is hoped that matters can be resolved to the parents' satisfaction.

Before referral there should be agreement between parents and school that the child does have a difficulty and that referral to the educational psychologist is necessary. In most cases this agreement exists but if the school is not in favour of referral then the parents are entitled to make their own referral to the Educational Psychology Service.

When the child is seen by the educational psychologist there should be an opportunity for the parents to discuss the findings, to ask any questions and to have clarified anything they are not sure about. Obviously if the parents suspect the child is dyslexic and the educational psychologist is of the same opinion all is well, but if she is not of this opinion then clarification is required.

There are a number of possible areas of disagreement. The parents may feel that insufficient *ASSESSMENT* has been carried out to warrant any conclusions being drawn. If they are happy about the assessment procedure itself then it is possible for there to be disagreement about the *CONCLUSIONS* arrived at. Also, it is possible that even if assessment and conclusions are agreed upon that the *RECOMMENDATIONS* made are a cause for concern.

Any disagreement should be settled as far as is possible by reference to the *facts* of the case rather than the feelings or opinions. Any parent could have a justifiable grievance if an inadequate assessment has been carried out, as it could be shown that certain areas of concern were not investigated – or at least not investigated fully.

However, if a full assessment has been carried out (one full enough to investigate all those areas of functioning giving cause for concern) then matters of disagreement rest on much narrower grounds. If, for example, the educational psychologist concludes that a child is *not* dyslexic but the parents think that the child is, then little progress is likely to be made by the parents simply stating their disagreement; they need to be able to show *why* they disagree. In these circumstances a firmly held belief *on its own* is insufficient to produce any changes; it needs to be backed up by hard facts. A solution usually found to be acceptable to all sides when these very rare cases occur is for the parents to be given a second opinion and arrangements for this can often be made by the first psychologist or the principal psychologist of the Service.

It is *possible* for there to be dissatisfaction with the educational psychologist's recommendations but this is not very likely if there has been agreement reached about the quality of the assessment and the conclusions drawn. It is possible for the parents to feel that insufficient help is being recommended initially and it is always possible that this can be amended to meet parental concerns after discussion with the psychologist. Even when parents and psychologist agree, there is still room for parental dissatisfaction at the next stage of the proceedings – that is, with the amount and type of special help offered by the LEA to the child concerned. Inadequate resources in all areas of education mean that those allocated to dyslexic children are constantly criticised along with the rest as being insufficient. Parents have every right to appeal to their LEA if they feel that their dyslexic child is not receiving adequate help, and should always do so.

The options parents have in the event of a grievance with any part of the assessment process is set out in more detail later (Chapter 12).

We now move on to look at possible causes of dyslexia. This requires two chapters as the topic is a lengthy, detailed one and the types of difficulty fall into two groupings: one connected with the *brain and visual system*, the other related to how a child acquires *phonic awareness* (knowledge of the individual sounds that go to make up words).

Chapter 9:
Possible Causes (I)
The Brain and Vision

Naturally, any parent of a dyslexic child wants to know *why* their child is dyslexic – exactly what it is that has caused their child to have the difficulty he does. Parents are not alone. Countless teachers, psychologists, researchers, etc., are also interested in knowing the answer.

Unfortunately the answer is not known. This is not for want of trying. Over the years since the condition was first recognised – and it is more than a century – there have been countless suggestions put forward. Some have been discounted but many remain in a limbo type of existence, neither proved nor disproved.

However, there are a number of lines of enquiry which appear to be more promising than others. They fall into two groups. One group of explanations is concerned with the manner in which the brain processes language and speech as well as visual and auditory perceptions. The other explanations are related to the way in which children are able to distinguish the different sounds which go to make up words (phonology).

This chapter and the one which follows are concerned with these two groups of possible explanations, brain functioning being dealt with here and phonology afterwards.

The Brain: Its Parts

The human brain is one of the least understood parts of the body and, although much more is known about it today compared with a century and a half or two centuries ago, our knowledge still answers only a very small fraction of the many questions that can be asked. In many ways it is as remote from us as the moon.

The brain controls virtually all the *activities* of the body – the movement of toes, feet, legs, fingers, hands, arms, eyes, head, jaw and tongue. It also controls those activities which take place without any thought or intention, such as breathing and the beating of the heart. In addition to all this the brain interprets the *information* about the outside world which is constantly being delivered to us through our eyes, ears, taste buds and senses of smell and touch. Information also comes to our brains through other, less well-known, senses e.g. balance, body movement and general body awareness. A third type of work undertaken by the brain is to produce the thoughts, feelings and emotions, together with the many other aspects of a person's detailed and complex personality. Strongly linked to the thought processes are those of communication. Language, of course, is part of this and reading, in turn, is a part of language.

To look at an actual human brain, or even a photograph of one, tells us very little about it. It looks rather like a large mushroom or a lump of drab, grey porridge without any distinctive shape, colour or other features. The surface is covered in ridges and clefts produced by the brain's surface being arranged in a series of folds. The medical term for a ridge is a gyrus (plural = gyri) and that for a cleft is a fissure (in the case of a deep one) or sulcus (plural = sulci) (for a shallow one). Figure 9.1 shows the brain in position seen from a viewpoint to the left, above and towards the back.

The main feature of the brain is that the surface is divided into two equal-looking halves by a fissure (the longitudinal fissure)

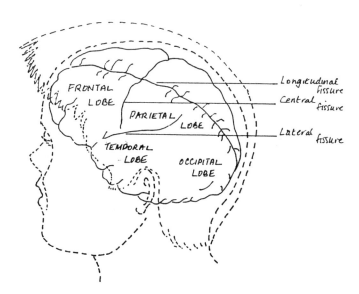

Figure 9.1 The brain - showing the main surface areas of the left cerebral hemisphere

running from front to back. The two halves are known as cerebral hemispheres and the drawing shows all of the left cerebral hemisphere and part of the right. One hemisphere appears as the mirror-image of the other. Each hemisphere is divided into four lobes. The central fissure separates the frontal lobe from the remainder and the lateral fissure separates off the temporal lobe (which is close to the ear and temple). At the rear top is the parietal lobe and at the extreme back is the occipital lobe.

We can learn more about how the brain is constructed by studying its appearance when it is cut through in various places. From the outside it looks as if the longitudinal fissure divides the brain completely into two separate hemispheres but in fact this is not so. The fissure descends so far and then ceases; underneath it the two halves of the brain are joined together. The means by which they are joined is a massive bridge of brain fibres known as the corpus callosum. This is shown in Figure 9.2 (one illustration from the side and one from the front). The corpus callosum does much more than merely join the two hemispheres of the brain together. The brain can function normally only if the two halves can communicate, i.e. can pass 'messages' from one half to the other. It is through the corpus callosum that these countless sensations which occur every minute are communicated from left side to right and vice versa. Differences in the size and form of the corpus callosum are found between people and give rise to different abilities. People differ in their mental

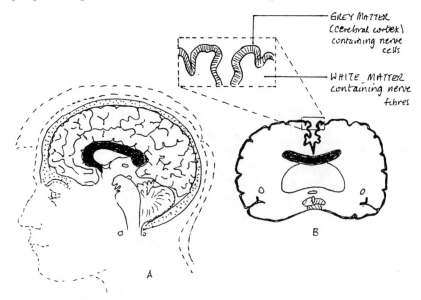

Figure 9.2 The corpus callosum (in black) viewed from the left side (a) and the front (b)

abilities because their brains grow in different forms. Males tend to differ from females, left-handers from right-handers and engineers from musicians.

Cutting through the brain also reveals the fact that the grey colour seen on the outside is not continued throughout but exists only as a thin (3mm) outer layer or covering. This is the cerebral cortex. Underneath this grey matter is the white matter. It is also seen that the brain is not solid throughout but has a number of cavities (known as ventricles) within it.

If a very thin section of the brain's cortex is taken and examined under a microscope it can be seen to be composed of large numbers of nerve cells – more than one million million of them (1 000 000 000 000) altogether. Each one of these can be connected up to as many as 25 000 others (the average being 10 000) and so the total number of connections in the entire brain is about 10 to the power of fifteen. This number is written in mathematical shorthand as 10^{15} and is so enormous that it represents two hundred thousand times the human population of the earth. The numerous foldings of the surface of the brain serve to increase its surface area and hence the number of nerve cells that can be accommodated there. This is shown on the right of Figure 9.2 and is labelled 'B'.

How the Brain Functions

The brain controls the body by means of 'messages' in the form of nerve impulses being passed from the cerebral cortex to the appropriate part of the body. An impulse reaches its destination by travelling down long nerve fibres. The messages/impulses consist of very small electric currents which are produced by changes in the body's chemicals. The nerve fibres involved act in much the same way as does an electric cable in the home when it carries an electric current to a light bulb or vacuum cleaner after the appliance is switched on.

The nerve fibres to, say, the foot, descend from the brain's surface down through the body of the brain and into the top of the spinal cord. They descend down to a particular part of the spine, at which they leave and travel down the leg to the foot. However, before they leave the brain the fibres *cross over* to enter the spinal cord on the side opposite to the cerebral hemisphere from which they originate. This has now transferred the nerve impulse to the *correct* side in relation to the foot concerned. The left side of the brain controls the right foot and vice versa. In fact, the working of the brain is such that the *right* hemisphere controls the *right* side of the *head* (affecting the eye and mouth movements) but the *left* side of the *body*. Toes, feet, legs, fingers, hands and arms are all controlled by that half of the brain which is on the opposite side of the body from them. For this reason the victim of a stroke located on the right side of the brain will have the right side of the face affected but the left arm and left leg. (This situation is illustrated in Figure 9.3).

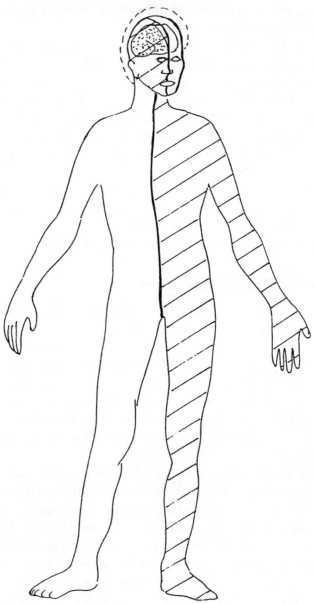

Figure 9.3 Parts of the body controlled by the right half of the brain

Despite this, however, it is not correct to say that the two halves of the brain are equal and identical in all respects, each doing exactly the same work as the other but on opposite sides of the body. Some of the functions carried out by one hemisphere are quite different from those of the other.

It is thought by some that there is probably an inborn tendency for the two hemispheres to develop differently and for the differences to increase over time through a person's experiences and the general learning processes. The two hemispheres are not equal partners in the organisation of movement – the left is the dominant one, for the vast majority of people at least.

The same is true for speech. The left hemisphere keeps the store of learned skills, programmes most movements *and also directs the right hemisphere* to control the left side of the body while it (the left hemisphere) keeps control of the right side. If the great mass of nerve fibres passing through the corpus callosum is divided, the movements of the right limbs (controlled by the left hemisphere) remain normal but movements of the left limbs become abnormal in a strange way. The person affected cannot comb his hair properly, accurately point the way or trace a circle on the ground with his foot. More automatic movements such as standing and sitting can be carried out quite normally, however. Injury to the right hemisphere will cause some paralysis of the left limbs but has no effect on the right limbs.

The Brain and Language

Each activity a person carries out is controlled by one particular area of the brain, and this area will be interacting constantly with other areas as appropriate. The two halves of the brain perform different tasks from one another but also communicate with one another.

In many activities the two halves do *not* have equal control of a particular activity but instead one half will take on most of the responsibility for the activity, forcing the other half to have a very much reduced part to play. The most powerful hemisphere is known as the DOMINANT one for the particular activity concerned.

Language is one activity of human beings which is controlled for the most part by one side of the brain. In the case of *most* people their language is processed mainly on the left side with the lesser amount of processing being carried out on the right. (Unfortunately the situation is not a straightforward one and that is why we emphasised that what we said can be claimed to apply to *most* people, but not all.

There are some people – a minority – who are different.)

Language figures strongly in our interest in relation to dyslexia as reading concerns the ability to interpret those symbols which represent language. In learning to read, a child must be able to master many skills such as hearing and understanding speech, seeing and perceiving both handwriting and print, speaking (for reading aloud) and writing. Figure 9.4 shows those particular areas of the left hemisphere which are concerned with the many skills involved in reading etc. as well as the manner in which two or more relate in the more complex activities.

A number of researchers believe that dyslexia can be explained, at least in part, by the situation relating to dominance. In most people while they are engaged in any activity related to language the left side of the brain plays a leading role. It is felt that dyslexia could result if the language areas are more or less equal in size as in this case there is evidence to suggest that a greater number of messages need to be passed from left to right across the brain through the corpus callosum. This results in the dyslexic person needing *more time* to understand what is being said to them or what they are reading. Similarly, more time will also be required to express themselves when replying.

The Brain and Vision

The manner in which our eyes and brain work together to produce the sense of vision is one of the most remarkable features of the human body. We are heavily reliant on vision for survival as about 95% of our knowledge of the outside world comes to us through our eyes. By means of vision we can detect light and shade, colours, movement and depth. We are also able to interpret what we see about us by converting so many signs into meanings, and this is particularly so in the case of reading where meaning is derived from the printed or written word.

The whole process involved in the visual system is extremely complex and although it is not necessary for us to have a detailed knowledge of it, nevertheless a familiarity with the basic details will help a great deal. Our eyes respond to light rays, which is why we cannot see anything in a totally dark place. When we are in normal daylight or sufficient artificial light there are countless rays of light entering our eyes from many directions. The rays themselves are invisible and each one is extremely narrow. Light rays travel in straight lines unless they strike something which causes them to

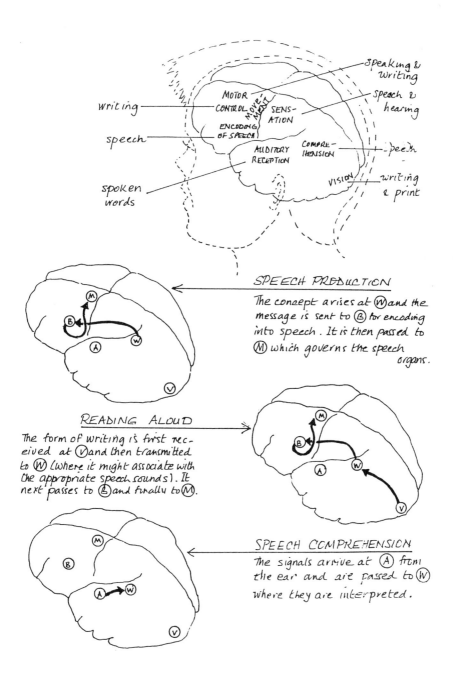

Figure 9.4 Language areas of the brain

change direction. Usually there are a number of rays found together and when this is so they form a beam.

We can learn something about how our visual system operates by considering what happens in just one of our two eyes when we are looking at an object somewhere in the centre of our overall visual field. (What happens in the other eye will be similar.)

The light rays pass from the outside world and strike the front of the eyeball. They pass through two layers (the CONJUNCTIVA and the CORNEA), a liquid (the AQUEOUS HUMOUR) the LENS, then a jelly-like substance (the VITREOUS HUMOUR), which fills most of the eyeball and finally make contact with the RETINA. All five substances through which the rays pass before reaching the retina are clear, colourless and transparent. By the time the retina is reached the light rays have undergone a number of distortions and changes of direction, the outcome being to place on the retina an image which is both upside-down and back to front in relation to the object itself. When the messages contained in the nerve impulses are passed from the retina into the brain it is necessary for the brain then to 'interpret' the messages, thereby making sense of the outside world by picturing it as it really is. (Figures 9.5 and 9.6 illustrate what we have said so far.)

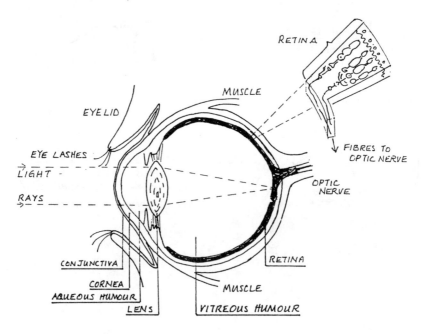

Figure 9.5 Structure of the eye

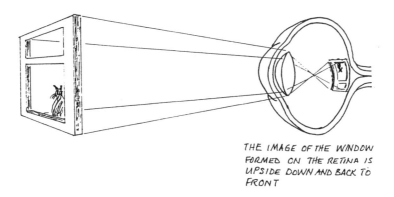

THE IMAGE OF THE WINDOW
FORMED ON THE RETINA IS
UPSIDE DOWN AND BACK TO
FRONT

Figure 9.6 Image formation in the eye

The Visual Pathway

This is the name given to the route taken by the nerve impulses as they travel from the eye through the brain to the right and left visual cortex at the rear.

The retina at the back of the eyeball is a light-sensitive layer consisting of a mixture of two types of cells (the **RODS** and **CONES**). The rods respond to differences in light and shade and the cones respond to different colours. The light rays must travel through the seven different layers of the retina in order to reach the light-sensitive part of the rods and cones.

When light falls on the retina it triggers a chemical reaction within the cells and this, in turn, converts into a nerve impulse that is passed out of the back of the eye by means of the two **OPTIC** nerves (there is one from each eye). These run backwards and towards each other, meeting at a particular point (the **OPTIC CHIASMA**) which plays a very important part in the process of visual perception. The optic chiasma is a crossing point. At this place nerve fibres cross over from one side to the other, but there is not a complete crossing over, only a partial one.

The nerve fibres which leave each retina in a bundle consist of two different groups, those from the left half of each eyeball and those from the right, but it is easier to consider them as belonging to either the outside (temporal) or the inside (nasal) half of each eye. What happens at the optic chiasma is that the fibres from the inside (nasal) half of each eye cross over to the *opposite* side of the brain and meet up alongside the outside (temporal) fibres of the other eye.

(*Note*: The optic chiasma is not to be confused with the corpus callosum as they are quite distinct. Although in each of these nerve fibres cross over from one half of the brain to the other, the optic chiasma is quite separate from the corpus callosum, being much smaller in size and located about $3/4$ inch (18mm) below the front of the corpus callosum. Another important difference is that in the optic chiasma there are only nerves related to vision whereas the corpus callosum contains a variety of different nerves.)

From the optic chiasma the two sets of optic nerves (now known as OPTIC TRACTS) continue to run back through the brain. The left optic tract consists of nerves from the outside half of the left eye and the inside half of the right eye. The right optic tract, in similar manner, contains the information gathered by the inside of the left eye and the outside of the right eye. The effect of this rather confusing-sounding arrangement has been to collect on the right side of the brain all of the information about the outside world which belongs to the left side of the total visual field, and vice versa. This produces a situation with which we are quite familiar – that of each side of the brain processing information which relates to the other side of the body (in this case the outside world closest to the other side of the body). (The total arrangement will be better understood by reference to Figures 9.7 and 9.8.)

Each optic tract enters another specialised area in the brain (a LATERAL GENICULATE NUCLEUS). From here nerve impulses are passed to different nerves (OPTIC RADIATIONS) which continue to pass back through the brain, eventually reaching the visual areas of the brain located in the occipital lobes.

This should give us some very rough idea of just how complex our visual system happens to be. Not only are the total mechanisms highly complicated, they are still not yet properly understood. The more complex a system is the more likely it is to have delicate parts and hence the greater the likelihood of something going wrong. Efficient vision relies on the efficiency of two eyes, each of which allows light rays to pass through and become distorted in the process, after which sense needs to be made of the distorted image.

Light energy at the retina is converted to chemical energy which in turn is converted into electrical energy. It is this which forms the basis of the nerve impulse passed from the retina through a series of nerve fibres to the visual cortex at the rear of the brain. The brain must then 'interpret' what the eyes have 'seen' in the outside world, whether it is a house, a tree, a car or a book.

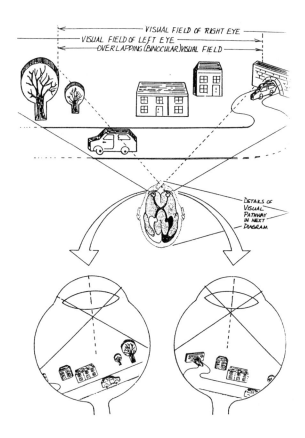

Figure 9.7 The fields and pathways for visual impulses

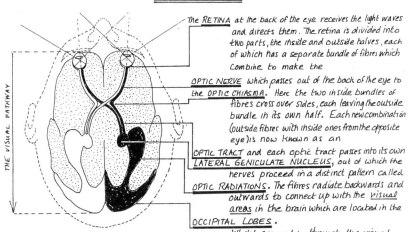

THE VISUAL PATHWAY

The RETINA at the back of the eye receives the light waves and directs them. The retina is divided into two parts, the inside and outside halves, each of which has a separate bundle of fibres which combine to make the

OPTIC NERVE which passes out of the back of the eye to the OPTIC CHIASMA. Here the two inside bundles of fibres cross over sides, each leaving the outside bundle in its own half. Each new combination (outside fibres with inside ones from the opposite eye) is now known as an

OPTIC TRACT and each optic tract passes into its own LATERAL GENICULATE NUCLEUS, out of which the nerves proceed in a distinct pattern called

OPTIC RADIATIONS. The fibres radiate backwards and outwards to connect up with the visual areas in the brain which are located in the

OCCIPITAL LOBES.

Whilst proceeding through the visual pathway the nerve impulses, conveying information about what the outside world looks like, have been organised in such a manner that information about the left half of the visual field is gathered on the right side of the brain and vice-versa.

Figure 9.8 The visual pathway

The fact that each retina contains 6 million cones and 120 million rods illustrates the extreme delicacy of the whole system. Also to be taken into account is the manner in which the eyeball can alter shape in order to focus images, as well as move about within the eye socket and scan the field of view. When what is being scanned happens to be a printed image from which meaning must be derived by also involving the language centres of the brain, a very complex situation becomes many times more so.

Because claims are made that dyslexia is caused by some inadequacy or malfunction in the eye–brain relationship we shall look at the commonest of these and consider how strong the evidence is.

Eye Dominance

Most people prefer one eye to the other such that they will always (or almost always) look through a telescope with one and not the other. The eye which is preferred on these occasions is known as the dominant eye and in the case of most people their dominant eye is on the same side as their preferred hand (the one they write with). Most people are right-handed and right-eyed. A child found to have his dominant hand and dominant eye on opposite sides of his body is described as 'cross-lateral' and some tests of dyslexia set out to investigate whether a child is cross-lateral or not.

Several investigators believe that eye dominance is important. When a child is looking at a distant object the line of sight of each eye is parallel and dominance has no part to play. But when looking at something close, such as a reading book, the sight lines converge and under these circumstances one eye becomes dominant.

Some people believe that dyslexia is associated with a failure to develop consistent eye dominance and so confusion results as to exactly where letters and words are on the printed page. It has been argued that more than half of the dyslexic population has an unfixed reference eye but the findings on which this claim was based have been criticised.

Other people are concerned that the muscles controlling fine eye movements are more important owing to the fact that during reading the eyes need to track across the page.

Eye Tracking

When we read something printed in English or many other written languages we must follow the line of print from left to right across the page. There have been reports of a high proportion of dyslexic people who tend to scan a line of print in the opposite direction.

If a dyslexic child tends to follow a line of print from right to left when in the process of being taught by a teacher who is not aware of this and who assumes that the child is tracking normally, then it is quite possible for the child concerned to develop a learning block associated with the printed word. (Reversals and some misreadings of words would also be explained by this difference.)

Competent readers are reported not to have a symmetrical visual scan. That is to say they do not 'take in' an equal number of letters to the right and left of any point on the page they are looking at. Rather, there are 14 letters to the right and only 7 letters to the left. Dyslexic children who do not possess this particular range and pattern of scan are obviously at a disadvantage.

There is little dispute that the eye movements of dyslexics when reading differ from those of normal readers but it is extremely doubtful whether this fact holds the answer to the problem of dyslexia.

Lenses and Filters

Some children report that they are able to read better if wearing spectacles fitted with specially tinted lenses or are reading a page through a coloured filter which overlies it. The use of these is closely associated with Helen Irlen of the Irlen Institute in the USA and reports of the successful use of lenses and filters have appeared in newspaper and television reports since late 1985. Helen Irlen claims that some people suffer from what she calls 'scotopic sensitivity syndrome' (or SSS for short), which refers to the ability to see when only low levels of light are available. However, there has been confusion caused, as a coloured filter will remove certain *wavelengths* of light but this is quite a different matter altogether from altering the *level* of light available.

Psychologists have attempted to test out the claims made for lenses and filters but this has proved to be difficult as many of the studies carried out (and on which the claims were made) have contained serious flaws. It was found in the various investigations that original studies suffered from shortcomings such as poor experimental design, lack of control groups, gains in reading being found to be quite low, reading tests being printed on coloured paper etc. Other investigations have shown that the lenses (of which there are more than 140 possible variations) acted mainly to absorb light rather than to cut out any particular wavelengths.

Researchers have found no greater degree of improvement in

dyslexic children's reading levels when using coloured overlays during reading than has been found in the case of other children. The evidence indicates that visual problems do *not* appear to be a major cause of dyslexia, and also that dyslexic individuals have only minor problems with *visual perception* but that they do have a difficulty in *recalling names* and with *'naming' language*. Difficulties of this type will be discussed in the next chapter.

The Brain and Hearing

The manner in which sounds heard reach and are interpreted by the brain is very complex but there are certain similarities to vision. Sounds coming into either ear set up nerve impulses to the brain but the nerve fibres that carry the impulses divide up so that some go to the half of the brain on the same side as the ear but the others go to the opposite half. However, each set of nerve fibres that *crosses over* is *stronger* than the set that stays on the same side. Hence, sounds heard in the right ear are interpreted for the most part on the left side of the brain and vice versa.

In most people language is interpreted by both halves of the brain but the left half has a larger language area than does the right and so is much 'stronger'. The right ear, for most people, is stronger when interpreting speech because it is more closely associated with the large language area in the left half of the brain. The left ear/right side of the brain is better at interpreting non-speech sounds.

It is thought that many severe dyslexics do not have their language areas sited mainly in the left hemisphere. If the brain, owing to incomplete dominance, must attempt to analyse language in both halves of the brain at once, the connection between the two halves through the corpus callosum could become overloaded and create confusion as to what needs to be interpreted. (Figure 9.9 summarises the situation.)

We are now able to move on in the following chapter to consider an entirely different type of possible cause(s) of dyslexia.

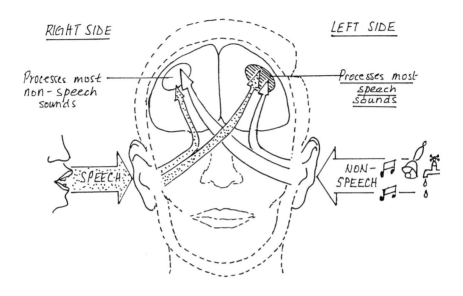

Figure 9.9 The brain and hearing

Chapter 10:
Possible Causes (II)
Phonemic Awareness

This chapter concerns a particular reading skill – *phonemic awareness.* The term will be explained later and the fact that a whole chapter is being devoted to it will be some indication of the degree of importance presently attributed to it in the field of dyslexia research.

The term relates to the sounds of our language and in order to understand the significance of it we need to spend some time discussing the heard and spoken aspects of language before we go on to relate it to the written form which needs to be read and which applies to dyslexia.

For the most part when we are in the presence of others we normally convey our thoughts and feelings by means of speech. Speech is usually delivered in chunks or units known as sentences, each of which makes sense. A sentence may be long or short, simple or complex but this is immaterial provided that it makes sense. Sentences are made up of words which can be quite short (one letter) or lengthy, and the words are found to be made up of syllables. Syllables in turn can be broken down into phonemes.

The relationship between words, syllables and phonemes can be understood by considering a few phrases. (The phrases are shorter than sentences but are sufficient for our purpose.) Our first example is:

a black dog

As we can see there are three words. However, there are also three syllables which we shall mark with a curved line for each:

a black dog

It is fairly easy to divide words up into syllables, as it is done by the pattern of speech sounds. A syllable is the smallest part of speech that normally occurs in isolation and has been compared to the beats that exist in relation to a piece of music.

The three words form three syllables because *'a'* is a vowel on its own and forms a single syllable, *'dog'* consists of a vowel with a consonant on either side and forms a single syllable and *'black'* is made up of a vowel at the centre with two consonants on either side. *Black* also consists of just one syllable. (Generally speaking there is syllable wherever there is a vowel – a, e, i, o, u – or a pair of vowels – ae, ai, au, ee, ei, etc. – or a y.) Now consider our second example:

a heavy cargo

This also consists of three words just as before, but in this expression there are *five* syllables:

a heavy cargo

'Heavy' provides two syllables, hea–vy in which *ea* acts as a single vowel and *y* also acts as a vowel. In the same way car–go provides another two. Because syllables are made up of phonemes there must be more of the latter than the former. Our first expression is found to contain eight phonemes and each will be indicated by a dot (.) below:

a black dog

This is almost a situation whereby each letter produces a phoneme but not quite, as *ck* produces only one sound, not two. In the case of our second expression the five syllables are found to be made up of ten phonemes:

a heavy cargo

The *ea* in 'heavy' combine to produce only one phoneme.

Phonemes

A phoneme is the smallest unit of sound that is present in a spoken word. A phoneme can be used to distinguish one word from another e.g. pin – bin, red – rod, leg – let. Phonemes are very important in speech and language as a change in just one of the phonemes in a word will alter the meaning of what is being said by producing a new word. The ability to read successfully depends very much on the learner reader knowing about the phonemes within a word – that is, on PHONEMIC AWARENESS.

Speech Sounds

Each one of the hundreds of thousands of words that go to make up the English language is made up of one or more phonemes. However, when the many thousands of words are analysed they are found to consist of various combinations of a much smaller number of basic sounds or phonemes – between 40 and 50, in fact.

The human vocal system is capable of producing many speech sounds but no one particular language ever makes use of all of them. There are speech sounds made by Chinese, Russians, Arabs and South American Indians which are never heard in English, and the converse is also true. (The scientific study of human speech sounds *generally* is known as PHONETICS and the study of how the sounds of *a particular language* are arranged in patterns so as to convey meaning is known as PHONOLOGY.)

In the case of English it is not possible for anyone to say precisely how many speech sounds are employed by the many millions of English-speaking people in the world when they are conversing together. An American, a Scotsman, a New Zealander, a Yorkshireman and a Cockney will all use slightly different speech sounds. In fact it is possible to claim that there is no such thing as *THE* English language but rather that there are a number of English languages, each of which has a large area of overlap with the others.

Because of this situation agreement was reached long ago as to what was to be regarded as correct and proper. This is usually called the Received Pronunciation (RP) of a language. Since the late 19th century there has been in existence an International Phonetic Alphabet (IPA) which was developed to produce suitable symbols for the sounds of any language. It has been revised from time to time, most recently in 1989. It is sufficiently rich to label the phonemes of any language and to handle the contrasts between them.

In the case of English there is a total of 44 phonemes in RP, 20 of them being vowel sounds and the others consonants. (These are given in Table 10.1.)

One of the things which an English-speaking child needs to learn as he grows is the manner in which the everyday speech he both listens to and uses comprises simpler sounds than words – the 44 phonemes. The child needs to know that a word is not just one 'block' of sound but is made up of a number of shorter sounds blended smoothly together to make one longer sound. The child must eventually learn that a word such a 'happy' consists of two 'beats' or syllables ha – ppy which in turn consists of a total of four phonemes h – a – pp – y (pronounced 'huh-ah-puh-ee') which, if written in the International Phonetic Alphabet, would be

h/æ/p/i

TABLE 10.1

THE PHONEMES OF THE ENGLISH LANGUAGE

Vowels (20)		*Consonants (24)*	
Symbol	*Sound (or value)*	*Symbol*	*Sound (or value)*
aɪ	try - wri<u>te</u>	b	<u>b</u>ack - ru<u>bb</u>er
aʊ	n<u>ou</u>n - n<u>ow</u>	d	<u>d</u>ay - ru<u>dd</u>er
ɑ	f<u>a</u>ther	dʒ	ju<u>dge</u> - Geor<u>ge</u> - ra<u>j</u>
ɒ	w<u>a</u>sh - <u>o</u>dd	ð	<u>th</u>is - o<u>th</u>er
æ	c<u>a</u>t - tr<u>a</u>p	f	<u>f</u>ew - pu<u>ff</u>
eɪ	d<u>ay</u> - st<u>ea</u>k - f<u>ace</u>	g	<u>g</u>ot - bi<u>gg</u>er
əʊ	g<u>o</u> - g<u>oa</u>t	h	<u>h</u>ot
ɛ	g<u>e</u>t	j	<u>y</u>et
ɛə	f<u>air</u> - squ<u>are</u>	k	<u>c</u>ar - <u>k</u>ey - clo<u>ck</u> - tre<u>kk</u>ed - <u>qu</u>ay
ɜ	h<u>er</u> - st<u>ir</u> - w<u>or</u>d - n<u>ur</u>se	l	<u>l</u>ip
i	h<u>e</u> - s<u>ee</u>	m	<u>m</u>uch - ha<u>mm</u>er
ɪ	sh<u>i</u>p	n	<u>n</u>ow - ru<u>nn</u>er
ɪə	h<u>ear</u> - h<u>ere</u>	ŋ	si<u>ng</u>
o	f<u>o</u>rce	p	<u>p</u>en - pe<u>pp</u>er
ɔ	n<u>or</u>th - w<u>ar</u>	r	<u>r</u>ound - so<u>rr</u>y
ɔɪ	n<u>oi</u>se - t<u>oy</u>	s	<u>s</u>ee - mi<u>ss</u>ed
u	l<u>u</u>nar - p<u>oo</u>l	ʃ	<u>sh</u>ip - mi<u>ss</u>ion
ʊ	f<u>oo</u>t - p<u>u</u>t	t	<u>t</u>en
ʊə	p<u>ure</u>	tʃ	<u>ch</u>urch - la<u>tch</u>
ʌ	b<u>u</u>d - bl<u>oo</u>d - l<u>o</u>ve	θ	<u>th</u>ree - hea<u>th</u>
		v	<u>v</u>ery
		w	<u>w</u>ill
		z	<u>z</u>eal
		ʒ	deci<u>s</u>ion - trea<u>s</u>ure

(Total = 44)

A further complication for the reading process is that the 44 different speech sounds are represented in print or writing by only 26 letters of the alphabet. Because there are insufficient letters to provide a one-to-one relationship with sounds the letters are used singly or in pairs to represent different sounds. Conversely, any one sound can be represented by different letters from one word to the next.

For example,	the *'oo'* sound in *shoot* is also
represented by	*ou* (in soup)
	u-e (in chute)
	ough (in through) etc.
Similarly,	the *er* sound in *her* is
represented by	*ir* (in sir),
	ear (in pear)
	air (in lair) etc.

These are only a few of the countless examples that exist. All in all, our alphabet of only 26 letters is thoroughly unsuited to the job it must do and the task of learning to read is not assisted.

At first, children are *not* aware of the individual phonemes that go together to make up a word. At a young age children are aware of only the *meaning* of a word or a sentence and it is only when they start to learn to read that they start to think about the sounds that are within words.

When young children are asked to imagine what a word would be like if one of its sounds was taken away (such as *train* without the *t* or *slip* without the *l*) they find the task difficult. It is only from an age of about eight that they can manage such a task quite well. Phonemic awareness is a skill which is obtained late in childhood.

Rhymes are a good example of phonemic awareness. If a child knows that *log* and *dog* rhyme then it means that he has broken down the words into *l-og* and *d-og* respectively and realised that there is the same *-og* sound at the end of each. The child who knows rhyme must know something about sounds coming together to form words. There is evidence to show that most young children are aware of rhymes, enjoy them and probably learn a great deal from them about the sound-base structure of their language.

The question arises as to whether young children who are insensitive to, and uninterested in, rhyme are likely to be dyslexic readers later in life when they are in school and attempting to master the skill of reading.

Research into Reading Difficulties

It is easy for anyone to make guesses as to why some children are poor at reading, but this is not good enough. What is needed is hard evidence. Countless times the question 'Why are some children dyslexic?' has been asked and reasons have been suggested but generally speaking most of the time people in the past *have not got it right*. Generally they have put forward reasons based on *inadequate evidence*. One investigator (Hinshelwood) claimed dyslexia to be caused by 'a difficulty in acquiring and storing up in the brain the visual memories of words and letters'.

If some particular difficulty within children were responsible for those children's reading difficulties then dyslexic children should, *in one specific way at least*, be quite different from other children.

What most researchers have done in the past is to have taken a group of dyslexic readers, given them a test in a particular skill (such as memory for words), compared the results with those from a matched group of non-dyslexic children and found that the dyslexics perform badly in comparison. The researchers have then *assumed* that the reading difficulties are *caused* by the poor skill involved.

On the face of it, of course, this appears to be a perfectly reasonable assumption to make but unfortunately there is a big snag involved. The snag is that in many cases the researchers have confused *cause* with *effect*. That is to say, the poor skill (such as poor memory for words) might be the *result* of not being able to read properly rather than the *cause* of it! In fact there are at least four situations which might exist in relation to the poor skill and the dyslexia:

(i)   The poor skill might be present in the child from early on, well before he goes to school and so might cause the dyslexia later.
(ii) The skill might develop poorly over time due to the dyslexia and so be a result of dyslexia.
(iii) The poor skill and the dyslexia might exist quite separately but happen to be present together in the same child (or children) by sheer coincidence.
(iv) The poor skill and the dyslexia might each be brought about by some third factor, as yet unknown to us.

As we said above, the majority of studies carried out have used control groups, the use of such groups being essential to the design of the study. Unfortunately the control groups have been used incorrectly as they have controlled inappropriate parts of the study. In comparing dyslexic with non-dyslexic children what has usually been controlled has been the size of the groups, the gender balance, the intelligence levels, the social factors etc. In other words, all factors likely to affect the outcome have been matched between the groups *except* the ability to read.

The criticism of these studies is that it can be quite misleading to compare such groups of children by means of *age* as the results will *not* tell the researchers what it is they are hoping to discover. If two groups, each of the same age and intelligence range, are matched then this is a mental age match. *But the groups need to be matched by reading age, not mental age, for meaningful results to emerge.* That is to say, there is nothing to be learned from comparing ten-year-old dyslexics who have a reading age of seven with ten-year-old non-dyslexics who read normally (i.e. have a reading age of ten years). What *should* happen is that the ten-year-old dyslexics should be compared with seven-year-olds who read normally (i.e. have a reading age of seven years also). This would place both groups, the dyslexics and the controls, at the same level of reading ability and would thereby produce a reading-age match instead of a mental-age match. If this were to be done and some differences *were* to be found, we know that it could *not* possibly be caused by a difference in reading levels as both groups are the same. Therefore the finding would be a significant one!

Having said that, the ideal type of research is difficult to carry out. Ideally the research would need to be carried out in three distinct stages in relation to dyslexic children:

1.   A 'reading-age match' type of study would need to be carried out, as just described. This would show that there actually was some genuine difference (such as a weakness in a particular skill) between dyslexic and other children.

2.   A large-scale study *carried out over a period of time* (likely to be some years in an investigation of this type) would be necessary in order to determine whether this particular skill weakness could *PREDICT* a future difficulty with learning to read.

3.   If the link between this particular skill weakness and future reading progress was found to be *strong* the weak skill would need to be improved by teaching and so demonstrate that when this occurs *so reading ability also improves.*

If something (which we shall call *x*) causes dyslexia than it must be present in a child *before* the child starts to make attempts at reading. It is hoped that it would be possible to detect *x* before the child embarks on the reading process, as described in point 2 above. This kind of study, because of the length of time involved, is described as *longitudinal* and would involve children being tested in the years before they begin to attend school and also being followed up for some years after they have been enrolled. A comparison of the test results obtained at the beginning of the study with success or difficulty in reading later on would show whether there is any relationship.

It needs to be said as a word of caution that any results obtained might not be as straightforward as might appear, as it is possible that both x and dyslexia are caused by a third unknown factor. Researchers must be constantly on the alert for this type of situation to arise.

Stage 3 above describes the technique to be used in order to get around this potential difficulty. Children need to be trained over a period of time in relation to x, the factor being studied. Naturally, a control group of children would be required, with this group not to be given any training. If the investigator is correct in her suspicions that x causes dyslexia then the 'trained group' should show an improvement in reading skills which the 'non-trained' group will not show.

By using experimental techniques such as those described briefly above, researchers have been able to produce two valuable types of results. First, they have been able to show that a number of long-held beliefs relating to dyslexia do not hold water. Second, they have been able to show that there *is* convincing evidence in relation to *phonemic awareness* for at least some of the difficulties faced by dyslexic children.

Taking the first-mentioned, strong doubts have recently been cast on the beliefs that dyslexic children:

*   produce mirror-image reversals when writing;
*   are particularly poor at perceiving or remembering shapes;
*   have greater difficulty with cross-modal perception (cannot relate the spoken with the printed word);
*   have greater difficulty in producing the correct word when they want to say something;
*   have poor memory for words.

Research into Phonemic Awareness

With regard to phonemic awareness (the main subject of this particular chapter) more and more attention has been paid over the last 20 years or so to children's awareness of the sounds that go to make up the words they hear and use every day.

One study (carried out in 1974) explored the difficulties children experience when attempting to divide up speech into phonemes. The young children, when given some examples of what was expected of them, showed that they could divide words up into syllables quite easily but found much greater difficulty in separating out the individual phonemes. *None* of those children aged about five were able to do the phoneme task; *less than 20%* of those aged about six were successful; and *only 70%* of the seven-year-olds were able to do what was required.

Since then, further research has shown a link between this ability to divide up words into phonemes (*phonemic segmentation*) on the one hand and *reading progress* on the other. For instance, children have been tested on their ability to find 'the odd one out' in a group of three or four words spoken to them. Sometimes the different phoneme was at the beginning of the 'odd' word:

bud – bun – rug – bus

sometimes in the middle:

mug – pig – dig – wig

and sometimes at the end:

run – but – gun – sun

The children tested were aged four or five and had not yet begun to read. When retested three or four years later there was a close relationship between the scores at four and five years and their reading ability when aged eight and nine. The same also applied to their spelling ability and this difference held true *even when allowances were made for differences in intelligence.*

Children who had made no progress in reading by the age of six but who were then given practice in *sounds* over a two-year period were found to make more progress in reading than similar children not given such practice.

In another study two large groups of children, one dyslexic and the other not dyslexic, were compared. The dyslexics did not do well at tasks which required both groups to detect and produce rhyme. This poor performance by the dyslexics resulted *despite* the fact that both groups were *matched by reading age,* i.e. the dyslexics were *older.* Also, the task involved only spoken and not written words. The dyslexics were found to be between three and six times worse than the controls. This is evidence of a definite and specific defect among dyslexic children. Although the dyslexics could actually read as well as the control group they were far behind in the ability to know whether groups of words rhymed or not.

Studies carried out in Sweden, the USA and England have shown that children who have a poor awareness of, and sensitivity to, rhyme during the years before they start on reading will not be able to read or spell as well as other children some years later. This finding holds true even when children of equal intelligence are compared. Furthermore, the finding holds good only for reading and reading-related skills such as spelling. It has no effect on success in mathematics, for example. What is more, the connection has been found to remain strong for as long as three years. It must be an important factor and other work has confirmed that this is so.

To people not constantly working with children who are learning to read and sometimes experiencing difficulties much of what has been said might be rather puzzling. It is difficult, for many adults, particularly ones who have never had reading problems themselves, to understand why a child should not be able to realise immediately that a word such as 'cat' when spoken is made up of three smaller sounds (which we will represent as kerr-urr-tuh). At first this is seems to be a very easy demand to make on a child, but it is not. Even when a young child is able to distinguish between 'cat' and 'cap' or 'cat' and 'mat' it is *still possible* for that same child to be completely unaware of the three segments/phonemes in each word and that there is only a one segment (or phoneme) difference between each pair. Those who believe that phonemic awareness (or, rather, lack of it) lies at the root of dyslexic children's difficulties claim that it is only when children begin to learn to read that they actually start to think about the small sounds within words. They claim that it is reading which produces an awareness of phonemes and not the other way about. To the dyslexic child words remain just words – indivisible and impenetrable. What is more, a dyslexic child may be unaware that written letters correspond to sounds, and even after being taught the fact will not find it easy to connect up a particular letter (or pair of letters) with the related sound.

A brief word should be said about SYNTAX as many feel that dyslexic children have difficulty with this also. Syntax is the grammatical (that is, correct) arrangement of words in speech or writing so as to make a sentence. It is bad syntax to say or write 'John was running along the road not looking where she was going' as the word 'she' should be 'he'. In the same way it is incorrect to say 'I am going to telephone Mary and speak to them' as 'them' should be 'her'. To have correct syntax in a sentence there must always be consistency with regard to gender, number and tense.

It is interesting to note that semantics (the meaning of words) plays no part in the difficulties shown by dyslexic children. Semantics is closely linked to intelligence but phonemic awareness is very much less so.

Irrespective of the exact cause, or causes, of dyslexia, a dyslexic child needs help. There is a variety of approaches to help a child overcome his dyslexic difficulties and a general picture of them is the subject of the next chapter.

Chapter 11: Help for the Dyslexic

During the century and more since dyslexia was first described, and particularly in the last 20 years or so, a considerable body of knowledge has been building up in relation to assisting the dyslexic child to read competently. Knowledge has also grown with regard to assisting in spelling, handwriting and other skills, and continues to do so. Older methods have also undergone revision and updating.

This chapter is intended to be as full a summary in the general sense as is possible. It is not possible in a work of this nature to go into great detail, the aim being to give an overview only.

There are a few general principles on which the overall work is based and these need to be mentioned at the outset. It is acknowledged that those children who are most severely dyslexic tend to make little progress with ordinary teaching methods. However, it is absurd to suggest that they are incapable of ever learning because they have failed to respond to these methods. (You will recall that in Chapter 7 the point was made that dyslexics do make progress over time, given the appropriate help.) However, dyslexic children do not all exhibit the same signs and symptoms, nor is any one symptom present in all dyslexic children to the same degree, so what will be an appropriate teaching method for one child will not necessarily be appropriate for another. The characteristics of the dyslexic are that the dyslexia can be severe, it is often very resistant to normal methods of remediation, and it may be accompanied by other difficulties, e.g. visual, auditory or motor. The typical dyslexic child needs to be taught on an individual or small-group basis and there are arguments to be put forward that certain children will respond best to one approach whereas others – those with different symptoms – will require something different.

Appropriate help for the dyslexic child in school is available in many forms and is brought to the child under a variety of different circumstances, so much so that there is a great danger of confusion arising in the mind of anyone, such as a parent, who is attempting to find out about the subject for the first time. Clear-cut, useful information on the matter is often difficult to obtain.

Any assistance available is part of the overall situation in which remedial provision is laid on for children and that assistance is, in turn, part of the very wide field relating to the normal teaching of reading throughout the country. Because of this there is a large collection of terms used, often with no common agreement as to what is meant by any particular one. Sometimes different terms are used by different writers to mean the same thing. Any parent attempting to find out what help is available is likely to be overwhelmed by such terms as reading scheme, programme, approach, technique, method, strategy, resource, procedure, system, etc.

An example will make this clear. One recent book describes ARROW, which stands for *A*ural - *R*ead - *R*espond – *O*ral – *W*ritten. The book says:

> This *approach* has been further developed by Lane (1990) under the aegis of the University of Exeter, School of Education in his ARROW *technique*. The *method* has its origins in infant teaching/learning approaches and was originally developed as a *technique* to help in the education of learning impaired pupils with marked difficulties in language skills attending a unit attached to a mainstream school.Children using the *system* will use at least one, and probably all, of the five components of ARROW.

The emphasis in italics is mine and was done to point out that even in these few lines ARROW has been described as an approach, a technique, a method and a system. In the normal course of events one would expect that the teaching approach would be something quite fundamental, indicating the particular direction, so to speak, in which the teaching would be directed. The approach having been decided, a programme would be planned out, starting at 'Stage 1' and moving through some number of other stages in a set order until the goal of full literacy were reached. Throughout the programme a number of techniques or methods would be employed, particularly if sticking points or places of difficulty were encountered and to assist in the overall task various aids and items of equipment would be employed.

If this is an acceptable description, then by broadening our viewpoint and looking at the overall situation relating to the dyslexic child we can see that there are five main factors that are involved:

- the TEACHER herself;
- the CONDITIONS under which the child and teacher meet;

- the general APPROACH followed;
- the particular TECHNIQUES or METHODS employed from time to time (within a more general PROGRAMME);
- the EQUIPMENT available to the teacher in her task.

The Teacher

All teachers must have basic teaching qualifications which for most newly trained teachers today means a university degree and a Certificate in Education, these two qualifications representing four years of full-time study. Those teachers employed to work with children with special educational needs tend to have at least one other qualification, this usually being a Diploma in Special Education which is awarded after a further full year of study.

The average remedial teacher (who might be called a specialist reading teacher, or support teacher, as titles vary from one LEA to another) will usually have a number of years of teaching experience, as the study for the Diploma in Special Education is usually undertaken only after some years of general classroom teaching. In LEA schools throughout the UK the teachers who provide specialist teaching for children with reading difficulties will obviously vary across a range when it comes to the number and type of qualifications they possess. They will also vary with regard to the number of years of teaching experience they have had and the type of pupils with whom they have gained their experience.

It will be a proportion of these specialist teachers who will be assigned or appointed to teach dyslexic children. Some, throughout the course of a working week, will be teaching only dyslexics, others will be teaching some dyslexics and some others with reading difficulties due to other causes. Some specialist teachers have had additional training in various approaches/techniques/methods that have been designed specifically to assist dyslexic children. There are many of these and a sample of 20 of them is given in Table 11.1. They represent most of the major approaches/techniques/methods that are presently being used in those institutions that specialise in identifying and helping dyslexic children.

As will be apparent, this sample of 20 was published, in the first instance, across a period of 47 years (from 1943 to 1990), during which time four of the earlier ones were revised, the latest in 1991. We have described them as approaches/techniques/methods because of the confusion about names which was explained earlier. As we can see, out of the 20 there are seven that are not given any description, three which are called *methods*, two *approaches*, two

Table 11.1: Samples of specialised teaching approaches

1. Fernald Multi-sensory Approach	1943	
2. Gillingham–Stillman Alphabetic Method	1956	
3. Edith Norrie Letter Case	1960	Revised 1970
4. Orton–Gillingham Method	1967	Revised 1987
5. Bannatyne's Colour Phonics	1967	
6. Alpha to Omega	1975	Revised 1990
7. The Hickey Method	1977	Revised 1991
8. Peabody Rebus Reading Programme	1979	
9. The Bangor Teaching Programme	1982	
10. Aston Index (Revised)	1982	
11. Aston Portfolio Checklist	1982	
12. Spelling Made Easy	1984	
13. Academic and Developmental Learning Disabilities	1984	
14. Children's Written Language Difficulties	1985	
15. Alphabetic Phonics	1985	
16. Tactics for Teaching Dyslexic Students	1986	
17. Dealing with Dyslexia	1986	
18. The Bangor Dyslexia Teaching System	1989	
19. The Icon Approach	1990	
20. Dyslexia: A Teaching Handbook	1990	

programmes, two *phonics* and one each of *system, tactics, checklist* and *index.*

The rate at which these approaches/techniques/methods grew in number shows an interesting trend:

> In the decade 1940–49 there was 1;
> In the decade 1950–59 there was 1;
> In the decade 1960–69 there were 3;
> In the decade 1970–79 there were 3 (+ 1 revision);
> In the decade 1980–89 there were 10 (+ 1 revision);
> In the year 1990 *alone* there were 2 (+ 2 revisions).

Recent years have produced a marked growth in the *rate* at which these approaches etc. have appeared and if the present trend continues the 1990s will outstrip the 1980s. (Figure 11.1 is a graph showing the trend.)

There are a number of points to be made about these approaches etc. in relation to the teacher. First, there are many available on the market and any specialist teacher is likely to be familiar with at least one and probably more. Second, the approaches etc. themselves vary a great deal in form and content. With some, all is explained in a manual but with others the teacher is required to attend a training course in order to become familiar with what is expected.

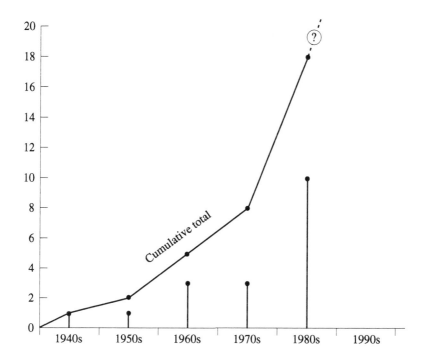

Figure 11.1 The growth of specialised approaches to overcoming dyslexia

The Conditions

The conditions under which a dyslexic child receives specialist teaching can vary tremendously across the board and will be influenced by a large number of factors, such as the LEA area in which the child lives, the particular school he attends, the general facilities available, the policy of the LEA on such matters, the wishes of the parents, the results revealed by the child's assessment, whether the child has been provided with a Statement of Special Educational Needs, etc.

The two major factors which underlie everything are the *amount of specialist teaching* provided to the child each week and the *setting* in which it takes place. A child might be taught for a comparatively short or lengthy total amount of time each week and the pattern of provision might be twice daily, once daily, twice weekly or some other. The child might be taught by one teacher or more than one and any particular teacher might be a staff member of the institution the child attends or a visiting specialist.

The child could be taught individually or in a small group (the size of which could vary from one situation to another), might be withdrawn from his class or be given support within it. It is also possible for the teaching to take place in the child's local school, or in a special unit or in a special school. If the special school happens to be the site where the teaching is provided then this could be either a day or a residential type. At the time of writing, in-class support would appear to be experiencing the greatest growth rate.

Other variations are also possible. The direct teaching of reading and other literacy skills is bound to be supplemented by various types of support. This may be provided at the systems level of the school so that teaching groups can be organised, the curriculum planned and teaching materials adapted. It could be that arrangements are made for two teachers to be available in the classroom (one always being available to assist a special needs pupil) or for parents to be available in a supportive role, or even for other pupils of the school to be assisting. Paired reading is often used and the precise means of doing so may take many forms, e.g. relaxed reading, shared reading, 'pause, prompt and praise', peer tutoring.

The Approach

It is possible to consider two types of approach which a teacher might make – general and special.

General approaches apply to most children in the course of learning to read and also to those with difficulties apart from dyslexia. Fortunately there are many approaches to reading which can be taken and it is part of the teacher's work to ascertain which is most suited to the child. This is bound to depend on matters such as the child's age, his reading attainments, his general intelligence, whether there are literacy difficulties *apart* from reading, what methods have so far proved to be unsuccessful and whether there are other factors involved, e.g. poor speech. Also, it is possible for a child to be taught by two or even more approaches at the same time.

Paired reading (mentioned previously) has been used with much success in many cases. In recent years computer-assisted learning (CAL) has developed greatly and now opens up many opportunities to many varieties of learning difficulties as well as dyslexia. The range and quality of the software available increases almost daily to assist not only with reading but also spelling (via the text processing) and handwriting (via the print-out facility). For well over two decades there has been a growth of publications in which the type of instruction advised for children with literacy difficulties has been linked to the results of individual assessments. These have *not* been designed specifically for children with dyslexia but nevertheless many dyslexic children have benefited. (Some indication of these are given in Table 11.2.)

Some approaches to teaching dyslexics are very much more specialised and we have already listed 20 of these earlier in this section (see Table 11.1). The majority of the specialised approaches concentrate on improving the child's ability to develop and use the phonic skills in which many dyslexics are at a disadvantage. Pupils with dyslexia need to be taught many basic skills that most children acquire quite easily. Whilst some believe in building up weaknesses, others concentrate on a child's strengths, and still more attempt both at once. In many cases dyslexic children are taught in exactly the same way as non-dyslexics but there is greater emphasis on such

Table 11.2: Materials linking assessment and teaching		
Early Detection of Reading Difficulties	Clay	1979
Preventing Classroom Failure	Ainscow and Tweddle	1979
Educational Applications of the WISC-R	Nicholson and Alcom	1980
Development of Reading and Related Skills with Pupils of Secondary Age (DORRS)	ILEA	1981
Barking Reading Project	Barking and Dagenham LEA	1982
Classroom Observation Procedure	ILEA	1982
Aston Index (Revised)	Newton and Thompson	1982
Aston Portfolio	Aubrey et al.	1982
Cloze Procedures and the Teaching of Reading	Rye	1982
DATAPAC	Akerman	1982
Linguistic Awareness in Reading Readiness	Downing et al.	1983
QUEST Screening, Diagnosis and Remediation Kit	Robertson et al.	1983
Special Needs Action Programme (SNAP)	Ainscow and Muncey	1984
Making Sense of It (Miscue Analysis)	Arnold	1984
Direct Instruction	Science Research Assoc	1985
Teaching with Precision	Raybuild and Solity	1985
Special Needs in the Primary School: Identification and Intervention	Pearson and Lindsay	1986
Learning Difficulties in Reading and Writing: A Teacher's Manual	Reason and Boote	1986
The Primary Language Record	Barrs et al.	1988
Early Identification of Special Needs	Wiltshire CC Ed Dept	1988
Bromley Screening Pack	Bromley LEA	1989
Touchstones	NFER	1989
Computer-assisted Learning Programmes with Speech Enhancement	Davidson	1990
Sound Linkage Programme	Hatcher	1994

matters as structure, detail, assessment, systematic teaching, over-learning and record-keeping. Ultimately, much time must be invested and there is no magic wand that can be waved, nor any kind of instant cure.

Programmes, Techniques and Methods

Very often a teacher will design an individual programme for a child which is excellent in principle and very much to be aimed at for any child with learning difficulties. However, there are also many commercially produced programmes available today which tend to be drawn on by teachers, as either entire programmes, or part of them, fit in quite well with what they feel the child requires.

The commercial programmes have a lot in common. The majority help the child to decipher print by using a phonic approach. To a greater or lesser extent they employ multi-sensory methods also. Programmes tend to be comprehensive and detailed and they often recommend a particular teaching order. The work is cumulative in so far as a typical programme will start with single letters and build up to words. Also, rote learning is considered necessary, as is overlearning.

Such programmes meet the characteristics recommended by the British Dyslexia Association that teaching should be:

- structured;
- sequential;
- cumulative; and
- thorough

Some commercially produced programmes are:

- Reading Recovery (1988) – developed in Ohio, USA;
- The English Colour Code Programmed Reading Course (1976)
- Patterns of Sound (1968)
- Pictogram System (1973)
- Signposts to Spelling (1978)
- ARROW (Aural – Read – Respond – Oral – Written) (1990)
- Attack-a-Track.

Some teaching techniques and methods of the many employed throughout the UK are:

- SOS (Simultaneous Oral Spelling);
- self-esteem enhancement;

- psycho-motor programmes;
- embedded pictures;
- mnemonic drawings;
- the use of tape recorders (often of special design);
- the use of plastic letters;
- finger spelling;
- syllabification;
- cursive script.

As will be apparent, techniques and methods are designed for one specific part of a programme – some to assist with just writing, others designed for spelling etc. There is a large measure of support for the view that no single approach, method or technique is appropriate for all dyslexic children at all stages in the development of their reading skills. It is unlikely that any two dyslexic children will experience identical approaches, programmes and techniques throughout the years of their school lives.

In 1990 a survey was carried out in order to seek the opinions of certain important organisations on a number of matters relating to dyslexia. Those contacted were:

The Department of Education and Science (DES) – since re-titled The Department for Education (DFE); The British Dyslexia Association; The Dyslexia Institute; The Dyslexia Unit at the University of Bangor; The National Association for Remedial Education; The Assistant Masters and Mistresses Association; The United Kingdom Reading Association; and NAS/UWT.

One of the aims of the survey was to discover which teaching approaches, programmes, techniques, methods or types of teaching assistance were recommended by each. The results were as given in Table 11.3.

Table 11.3: Types of approach and recommendations

Type of teaching approach/programme etc.	Recommendations (out of total of 8)
Multi-sensory	7
Phonics	4
Perceptual Training	4
Memory Training	3
Contextual Clues	3
Curriculum Support	3
Study Skills	3
Objectives	3

Others that were given mention were: support from specialist teacher, sequencing training, motor skills training, spelling rules, language skills, automaticity, number, enjoyment of reading and writing, word processing, use of tapes, letter-formation training, word recognition, reading strategies, writing strategies, metacognition, essay practice, paired/peer reading, behavioural skills and counselling.

(A number of other recommendations were made by the eight organisations and these were of a wide-ranging nature covering matters such as the training of teachers, the design of school buildings and the equipment which should be made available.)

Equipment

The basic equipment available to the teacher will be exactly the same as for any teacher so far as the dyslexic child can be taught by means of everyday classroom equipment, there being greater importance attached to the manner in which the teaching is done. The teacher and child should, therefore, have such items as a blackboard, access to a photocopier and books, including dictionaries, work books and work sheets.

There should also be relevant wall charts, letters of the alphabet available on cards (for example as in the Edith Norrie Letter Case), also those cut out of wood, those in plastic mould form, letters cut from sponge, rubber and either 'fuzzy felt' or magnetic ones (preferably both). A sentence maker and flash cards are likely to be required also.

Games that involve letters and words are very valuable to children with reading difficulties and so 'Scrabble', 'Snakes and Ladders', 'Lexicon' etc. should be available. Much can be learned even in a play situation. Information technology has recently brought what was formerly very expensive equipment well within the budget of schools and units. Nowadays it is quite commonplace for a school to have a tape recorder, audio-cassettes, portable typewriters, small electronic spelling machines, computers and word-processing equipment. Peripherals such as printers are also quite common. All of these can be used to advantage by a dyslexic child.

More specialised equipment also exists, some of it at reasonable cost. Triangular-sectioned rubber pencil grips benefit those with writing difficulties and are quite cheap. The Edith Norrie Letter Case referred to above has proved invaluable over the years since its introduction as has the SALVA machine (*See-And-Learn-Visual-Aid*).

Support Teaching

Having gone over very quickly the overall scene in relation to helping the dyslexic child, it needs to be said that most children are being assisted by remaining within their respective class and being given support teaching. This is a trend which is growing. There are many reasons for this which need not be detailed here, but generally the trend is for greater integration of children with special educational needs. A survey carried out in 1987 found 14 different forms of support for learning available in mainstream secondary schools and another survey in 1988 found a mixture of sets, withdrawal, support teaching and special classes. (Withdrawal and support teaching were the two most widely used). The general philosophy underlying the present approach to children with learning difficulties is that all members of staff should be aware of and attempt to assist these children's difficulties, that the children should be given access to the whole of the curriculum, that their learning should be supported, and if possible the curriculum should be differentiated for them, i.e. delivered at a level and pace appropriate to the learning difficulties they are experiencing.

Earlier in this chapter a brief description was given of the manner in which support teaching could be organised for a dyslexic child within the ordinary classroom and so there is no need to repeat it here. However, to give some details of the types of outcome of such support we can list the following:

- specially prepared work sheets;
- teaching any specialised vocabulary prior to a lesson;
- providing a tape recording of literature being studied;
- providing photocopied notes (to save note taking);
- arrangements to tape record notes etc.;
- arrangements for transcribing work from a tape recording;
- use of a word processor – including tuition;
- tuition related to work organisation;
- a remedial programme to overcome a specific weakness.

Obviously many of these will be of assistance to other children with difficulties, not just dyslexics. *We shall complete this chapter by setting down the PRINCIPLES on which the teaching of dyslexic children should be based:*

1. Teaching to be undertaken only after a full assessment of the child.

2. The diagnosis of the child's difficulties to be made as early as possible.
3. The general approach to be based on utilising strengths and minimising weaknesses.
4. Daily tuition for the severely dyslexic child.
5. All books etc. used to be stimulating and interesting.
6. Books etc. not to be those associated with previous classroom failure.
7. The vocabulary used to be controlled.
8. The teaching to be carried out with an individual child or a small group of similar children (although this teaching does *not* need to be on an all-day basis - see no.10).
9. All pressure to be removed from the child.
10. The child to remain with his or her intellectual peers in class and be withdrawn for regular, short spells of individual assistance).
11. Less written work to be expected than from others.
12. Class marks to be awarded on the basis of *oral* responses.
13. Dyslexic child to sit at front of class, not in the back row feeling neglected.
14. Dyslexic child to be given access to correct spellings.
15. Teacher to let child have his own alphabetically indexed notebook.
16. Teacher to let child do homework/classwork with text books open.
17. Dyslexic child not to stay on one book too long. After a while a book should be substituted for a different one at the same level.
18. Writing done on the blackboard always to be very clear.
19. Important new words to be written up clearly.
20. Teacher to avoid giving *long* lists of spellings to be learned, as small successes are better than total failures.
21. Like-sounding words (homophones) not to be put together.
22. Mistakes in written work should never be read out in front of whole class.
23. Emphasis should be placed on the child competing with himself, not others.
24. Withdrawal timetable to avoid impinging on favourite lessons.
25. A time *limit* for homework should be set.

The next chapter consists of various types of advice, all of which, it is hoped, you will find useful in attempting to gain assistance for your child. Most parents are not familiar with the law relating to special educational needs, nor are they always aware of what their rights and the rights of their child are. 'A guide through the maze' is required and the next chapter attempts to provide this service.

Chapter 12:
Advice for Parents

If our society was better organised than it actually is, then all dyslexic children would be identified early, assessed adequately shortly afterwards, be reported on in an efficient manner with their needs fully described and soon after that be provided with assistance of the correct type and quality to meet their needs. Unfortunately, real life is far short of what it could be and so this does not happen for all children.

The aim of this chapter is to provide advice for parents of dyslexic children, describing the difficulties that they might encounter at any stage of the process from when the suspicion of dyslexia first arises to that when assistance is eventually provided. Suggested courses of action are given for each possible point of difficulty. There are three main stages in the whole process, each of which can be spread over an indefinite period of time and also broken down into a number of smaller stages. These main stages are:

1.   when dyslexia is first suspected;
2.   the assessment;
3.   the provision.

Dyslexic children are children with special educational needs and must always, therefore, be dealt with by the same overall framework and general processes as laid down in law for all such children. We will briefly describe them so as to be familiar with the overall context in which all education personnel must operate.

The Department for Education (DFE) suggests that schools should attempt to meet a child's special educational needs (SENs) by embarking on a staged process. It is suggested that there could be as many as five stages altogether and the DFE has described these in a 134-page booklet entitled *Code of Practice on the Identification and Assess-*

ment of Special Educational Needs. The Code of Practice was published in 1994 and came into effect on 1 September of the same year.

The 1993 Education Act required the Secretary of State to issue this Code of Practice to all LEAs and the governing bodies of all maintained schools so that all concerned would be aware of what their responsibilities were with respect to children with special educational needs. Since it came into practice schools must have regard to it – they cannot ignore it.

That said, the Code can only offer guidance; it cannot and does not attempt to give every detail of what ought to be done in each individual case. Schools were not expected to have information on their SEN policies by 1 September 1994 nor to have set up procedures to match those set out in the Code. However, it was expected that schools would have these by 1 August 1995 and would afterwards report them to parents. Partnership with parents is an important principle in the Code. Where agreement cannot be reached parents have access to a quick and independent system of appeals against LEAs' decisions and a new SEN Tribunal has been set up to deal with these cases.

The Code sets out the criteria LEAs should use in deciding whether to carry out a statutory assessment, and part of the Code (pages 56–58) deals with: *Specific learning difficulties (for example Dyslexia).* It describes some children who 'may have signficant difficulties in reading, writing, spelling or manipulating numbers, which are not typical of their general level of performance'. It identifies them as being able to gain some skills in some subjects quickly and having a high level of oral ability yet encountering sustained difficulty in gaining literacy or numeracy skills. It goes on to state that the LEA 'should seek clear, recorded evidence of the child's academic attainment' and then ask certain relevant questions relating to:

(i)   discrepancies in attainments;
(ii)   expectations on the part of teachers etc. which are above attainments;
(iii)   evidence of clumsiness, difficulties in sequencing or visual perception, deficiencies in working memory or delays in language functioning;
(iv)   severe emotional and behavioural difficulties, an inability to concentrate, frustration or distress in relation to learning difficulties etc.

The Code goes on to set out other questions the LEA should ask, these relating to the action taken by the school up to that point. These questions concern matters such as:

(i)   how the curriculum and the school day have been made *accessible* to the child;
(ii)   what *individual education plan* has been formulated/monitored/ evaluated; for example, for *reading*, for *spelling* and the use of *multi-sensory teaching strategies*;
(iii)   whether the child's progress has been *monitored*;
(iv)   to what extent the parents have been involved;
(v)   the use of appropriate information technology;
(vi)   whether attempts have been made to reduce anxiety and enhance self-esteem;
(vii)   whether the school doctor's or family GP's assistance has been sought.

The section relating to dyslexic children finishes by describing the circumstances under which a statutory assessment should take place. These are if the child's difficulties are significant and/or complex, have not responded to appropriate measures and are of such a nature that they *may* require a special type of provision (which could not reasonably be expected to be available within the ordinary school).

The thinking behind the document is quite clear. The DFE expects all schools to go through a set procedure for every child suspected of having special educational needs in the belief that this will ensure a thorough assessment of the needs of each child. (It will also go some way to making the assessment process uniform from one LEA to another.)

The DFE also works on the basis that all children with special educational needs, when considered together as a group, will show great variation from one to the other. There will be a gradient with children who have quite mild needs at one end, progressing through an ever-increasing continuum to severe, multiple and complex needs at the other. The DFE, therefore, expects each child to be 'matched up' to the correct type and quantity of extra assistance that is appropriate for his (or her) individual case. The five suggested stages are set out in Table 12.1.

What these stages mean, in practical terms, is that once a school identifies a child as a cause for concern then the school should do its best to see if it can meet the child's needs from within its own resources. If this is tried for an appropriate period of time and found

Table 12.1: Stages, action and agency in the provision of assistance to the child with special educational needs

Stage	Action	Agency
1	Class or subject *teachers*: • identify a child's special educational needs • consult the school's SEN coordinator • gather information • take initial action	School
2.	The school's *SEN coordinator*. • takes lead responsibility for managing the child's special educational provision • works with the child's teacher	School
3.	Teachers and the SEN coordinator are supported by *specialists from outside the school*	School
4.	*The LEA*: • considers the need for a statutory assessment • makes a multi-disciplinary assessment if appropriate	School and LEA
5.	*The LEA*: • considers the need for a Statement of Special Educational Needs • makes a Statement if appropriate • arranges provision • monitors provision • reviews provision	School and LEA

not to be effective then a specialist teacher or other relevant person should be called in to advise, and the school should act on that. In the event of this not being successful, referral needs to be made to the Educational Psychology Service so that the school's educational psychologist can assess the child and also give appropriate advice.

Should the psychologist feel that the child would benefit from a full multi-disciplinary assessment she will inform the LEA of her opinion and the LEA will decide whether to proceed with this. In the event that they do so they must finally consider all the evidence presented to them and decide whether the child has difficulties which are severe and/or complex etc. (as described earlier in this chapter).

If the LEA decides that the child does fall into one or other of these two categories then it must issue a 'Statement of Special Educational Needs' in which the child's needs are described and also the provision which is going to be laid on in order to assist in meeting

those needs. The school or unit where it is intended the needs shall
be met is also to be included. (The Statement is aimed at safeguard-
ing the child's rights to be provided with something different or
extra. Once issued the provision *must* be laid on and the child's right
to such provision is legally protected). The Statement cannot be
amended or withdrawn without sound educational justification. The
child should be monitored and reported on, at least annually. In the
light of the findings the Statement must then be reviewed with pro-
visions amended as appropriate. That is to say, the LEA must increase
the provision if the level is found to be insufficient but can also
decrease it, or even terminate it if it is felt that such is justified. Any
changes must be noted in the Statement and when it is felt that extra
provision is no longer required then the Statement is withdrawn.

So much for the theory. As will be appreciated, the *Code of Practice*
is set out in very general terms because it applies to all children with
special educational needs, not just dyslexics. Children with SENs
form a very wide-ranging group and display many types of difficulty.
Most of these can be present in a child in varying degrees as well as
in various combinations. It is generally held that 20% of children will
have special educational needs at some stage during the 11 or more
years of their statutory education but that only 2% will have needs
that are sufficiently serious to justify the provision of a 'Statement'.

We must now consider each of the three important stages we
mentioned at the beginning of the chapter. (These are not to be
confused with the five stages of assessment given in the *Code of Practice*).

When Dyslexia is First Suspected

A number of problems can arise in the case of any dyslexic child, as
any parent will appreciate. In the first place many dyslexic children
come to the attention of parents and teachers as having difficulty
with reading and so it can often be difficult, depending on the
circumstances, to distinguish the dyslexic child from others who are
generally slow. It could well be some time before the true nature of
the child's reading difficulty becomes known. Another possible problem is that it could be the parents, rather than the school, who first
suspect dyslexia and in this case they will need to bring their suspicions to the head teacher's attention. Whoever first suspects dyslexia
is not important. What *is* important is that the suspicions must be
shared immediately – parents with school or school with parents. At
this stage, it is the communication that is vital in order to speed up

getting help to the child, as well as home–school cooperation.

Generally speaking matters are probably more likely to proceed in a straightforward manner if the school is first to suspect dyslexia and then informs the parents, as in these circumstances parents tend to cooperate fully in what the school suggests. However, if it is the parents who first bring their suspicions to the school it is more likely that misunderstandings or delays could arise. In most cases the school will do all it can to allay parents' worries and meet their wishes, but sometimes the school will not be of the same opinion as the parents, or feel that the evidence available is not strong enough for such suspicions, or even believe that the parents are over-anxious. It could also be the case that the school would like further time to work with the child before reaching a decision as to whether dyslexia is involved.

Preferably, it will require only a discussion between parents and head teacher to produce agreement on both sides about what is to be done and the timing of such action. If, for whatever reason, it is not possible for parents and school to agree on the nature of the child's difficulties, then the matter can easily be resolved by referring the child to the educational psychologist. Should the school be reluctant to refer the child it is quite in order for the parents to make the referral themselves. Should this action on the parents' part happen to result in a situation they find unsatisfactory then it is possible to contact the principal educational psychologist.

Of course, the school and parents could be in complete agreement that dyslexia is the cause of the child's difficulties but the school might consider it unnecessary to refer to the educational psychologist. The school might feel that the severity of the problem is not as great as the parents believe it to be, or that the child can be helped sufficiently from within the school's own resources. Obviously parents should carefully consider what the school has to say on the matter but if, in the final analysis, there is disagreement then the parents are quite entitled to make the referral themselves.

The Assessment

When, by whatever means, the educational psychologist is brought into contact with the child there are some aspects of the process which might cause parental concern or at least give rise to questions. It is to be hoped that the child will be seen shortly after referral or at least without too long a delay. If the educational psychologist has a lengthy waiting list there is little that can be done except to request that some priority is given. This might result in an earlier referral particularly if the parents are willing to accept an appointment at short notice resulting from a cancellation.

Of more importance, of course, is the actual assessment itself (including the results, the psychologist's interpretation and the recommendations). The parents should be satisfied that the assessment was sufficiently thorough as to properly investigate the child's difficulties, describe them accurately and lead to some conclusions being drawn. Some impression will be gained from what the psychologist says in interview afterwards, but the parents can only *act* on what is contained in the written report.

If a parent feels that the assessment was not sufficiently thorough, then a request can always be made for the psychologist to do further investigation. If the parents are unhappy about the actual findings because, for instance, they do not conform with what they themselves know about their child, then it is always possible to request a second opinion. The same applies if the parents agree with the findings but not with the recommendations. For instance, if the psychologist does not feel that the child should undergo the 'Statementing' procedure but the parents wish for it to happen then an appeal is also possible in this situation.

The Provision

Dyslexic children vary considerably from one to another, particularly in the degree to which they are affected, so it is not possible to discuss the provision for such children in more than vague terms. What also complicates the overall picture is that the provision available for dyslexic children varies from one LEA to the next, and even between schools within the same LEA.

What is important is that any particular dyslexic child gets assistance of the correct type and quantity to result in that child's difficulty being adequately remedied *irrespective* of whether a 'Statement' has been issued or not. After the child's needs have been adequately assessed, and the necessary help agreed on, then that help *must* be provided. As part and parcel of the same process, regular reviews of the child's progress need to be carried out so as to ensure that what is being provided is effective. If parents feel that provision is inadequate or inappropriate then they have the right to ask for their child's situation to be reconsidered.

Figure 12.1 summarises the stages that a dyslexic child with a significant degree of difficulty is likely to go through before being provided with a 'Statement of Special Educational Needs' by his

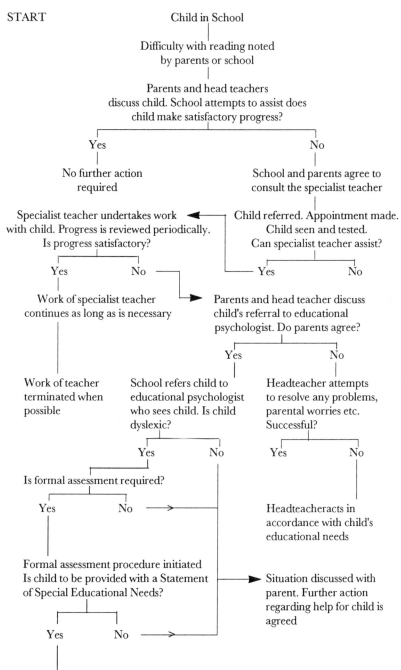

START   Child in School

Difficulty with reading noted
by parents or school

Parents and head teachers
discuss child. School attempts to assist does
child make satisfactory progress?

Yes   No

No further action
required

School and parents agree to
consult the specialist teacher

Specialist teacher undertakes work
with child. Progress is reviewed periodically.
Is progress satisfactory?

Child referred. Appointment made.
Child seen and tested.
Can specialist teacher assist?

Yes   No   Yes   No

Work of specialist teacher
continues as long as is necessary

Parents and head teacher discuss
child's referral to educational
psychologist. Do parents agree?

Yes   No

Work of teacher
terminated when
possible

School refers child to
educational psychologist
who sees child. Is child
dyslexic?

Headteacher attempts
to resolve any problems,
parental worries etc.
Successful?

Yes   No   Yes   No

Is formal assessment required?

Yes   No

Headteacheracts in
accordance with child's
educational needs

Formal assessment procedure initiated
Is child to be provided with a Statement
of Special Educational Needs?

Situation discussed with
parent. Further action
regarding help for child is
agreed

Yes   No

Extra educational resources assigned to meet child's special educational needs. Progress
kept under formal annual review. Statement is *EITHER* maintained until child leaves
school (which could be at age l9 years). *OR* is withdrawn when considered appropriate.

Figure 12.1

LEA and the given the necessary help. (The flow diagram also includes details relating to a child whose difficulties are less serious.)

It would be incorrect to assume that the general situation is a pessimistic one and that assessment and help will never be provided for a dyslexic child unless the parents embark on a lengthy and bitter battle with their LEA. Quite the opposite is the case, in fact. Over time teachers and their LEAs have become more aware of dyslexia, its prevalence and the need for resources to assist with it. More children are being recognised, assessed, diagnosed and recommended for specialist help. More teachers are undergoing the necessary training to be able to provide the requisite expertise necessary to assist. As time progresses the situation for dyslexic children is seen more and more to be one of constant improvement.

Of course, the rate of improvement in the situation is not as rapid as parents would wish and needs are not yet being fully met but the overall situation at present is definitely an improvement on that of some years ago. The aim of this chapter is to provide guidance to those comparatively few parents who *might* encounter some difficulty at *some* stage. It is not thought that all or even most parents will face any serious problems. (For those who find it useful, the whole process has been summarised in Table 12.2).

Parents' Rights

At the present time parents have far more rights with respect to their children's education than ever before. When a child has special educational needs parental rights become particularly powerful and far-reaching.

It is probably worthwhile to set these out in detail, as not all parents are aware of just what rights they have when problems arise with their child's educational progress such that assessment is required and special educational needs are diagnosed. It is also worth knowing that there are many independent agencies that a parent may turn to for advice and support if they encounter difficulties when attempting to gain help for their dyslexic child. Different rights apply to different stages in the assessment procedure and so have been gathered together accordingly in the list which follows.

Parents' rights in relation to their child's special educational needs and the assessment of those needs under the 1993 Education Act

Parents have the right:

When choosing a school...

Table 12.2: The resolution of parents' grievances

Area of concern	Possible action
Parents concerned that a child has reading difficulties but concern not shared by school	Seek the advice of the SEN teacher. If still concerned seek the advice of the educational psychologist
School shares parental concern about lack of progress but feels dyslexia not the cause	Request an educational psychologist's opinion. If any difficulty encountered, contact the principal educational psychologist
Parents and school agree about likelihood of dyslexia. Parents request referral to educational psychologist but school reluctant to do so	Write to the principal educational psychologist and request an assessment of child's special educational needs. If a difficulty still remains then write to the Chief Education Officer summarising events and repeating the request
Child assessed by educational psychologist but parents unhappy about the nature of the assessment (e.g. not thorough)	Discuss with educational psychologist and request further assessment. If this does not resolve matters contact the principal educational psychologist
Parents satisfied with the nature of the assessment but disagree with the findings, e.g. they contradict what parents feel	Discuss with the educational psychologist. If the matter unresolved a second opinion can be requested via the principal educational psychologist
Parents satisfied with nature of assessment and findings but not with the conclusions reached (e.g. child not dyslexic)	as above
Parents satisfied with nature of assessment, findings and conclusions but not with the educational psychologist's recommendations (e.g. child does not require any extra support)	as above
Parents satisfied with the assessment by the educational psychologist but not with the LEA decision (e.g. not to issue a Statement)	Appeal against the LEA decision
Parents agree with LEA about the need to issue a Statement but disagree with the type of provision proposed	as above
Parents agree with Statement being issued and with the type of provision proposed but disagree with the amount of provision	as above

1. ...to obtain in writing general information about the range of special educational provision available within their LEA. (Each LEA produces a booklet which is updated annually).
2. ...to obtain in writing specific information about a particular school or schools. (Each school produces a booklet which is updated annually).
3. ...to visit any school to ask questions etc.

In assessment procedures...

4. ...to request an assessment of their child at any stage.
5. ...to make a complaint if this request is refused and they consider the refusal to be unreasonable.

For children under five (not relevant in the case of dyslexic children)...

6. ...to refuse an LEA request for an assessment if their child is under the age of two years.
7. ...to be informed by the Health Authority if it considers that their child under five has special educational needs.
8. ...to obtain from the Health Authority information about any voluntary agency which it believes might be able to help them.
9. ...to be advised by their LEA, if their child is under two, of the best way of helping their child (e.g. nursery provision etc.).

If the LEA requests an assessment...

10. ...to early consultation and full discussion about their child's difficulties.
11. ...to have their views and feelings taken into account (i.e. be given an opportunity to put them in writing and have them circulated to concerned professionals).

If the LEA decides to go ahead with assessment...

12. ...to have explained to them the procedure which is to be followed.
13. ...to be given the name of someone in the LEA who can be contacted for more information.
14. ...to be given 29 days in order to make a 'representation' to the LEA (i.e. be given the opportunity to tell the LEA whether or

not they agree with the decision and to gather any reports etc. in support).

When the assessment is being made...

15. ...to attend any interview their child has.
16. ...to expect that relevant professionals are supplied with a copy of their representations.
17. ...to be informed of the purpose of any examination, also where and when it is to take place, how to get more information and how to make their views known.
18. ...to refuse permission for a move to another school for a short period.

After the assessment...

19. ...to be informed, in writing, of the LEA's decision whether to produce a STATEMENT OF SPECIAL EDUCATIONAL NEEDS.
20. ...to be given a draft version of the Statement for their comments.
21. ...to be given an accompanying copy of all reports and evidence submitted by the various professional advisers.
22. ...to ask for a meeting with the LEA to clarify anything they are unsure of, etc. (This request is to be made within 15 days).
23. ...to request a further meeting after this one in order to question any of the professionals. (This request must be made within 15 days of the first meeting).
24. ...to put their final comments about, and criticisms of, the Draft Statement to the LEA and also to make their own alternative proposals.

Getting help...

25. ...to consult their own advisers and get a second opinion from, for example, The Panel of Independent Experts on Special Educational Needs.

The Statement of Special Education Needs...

26. ...to appeal against the LEA decision not to produce a Statement if they believe one should be produced.

Appealing against the Statement...

27. ...to appeal against the Statement or any part of it if they feel there is justification in doing so.
28. ...to be given 14 days notice of the time and place of the appeal and for it to be held in an accessible place at a convenient time.
29. ...to have a friend or representative at the hearing of the appeal.
30. ...to have witnesses at the appeal.
31. ...to submit written statements from experts.

The appeal...

32. ...to be informed in writing of the decision.
33. ...to appeal in writing if still unhappy.
34. ...to complain if they feel that the behaviour of the appeal committee was unfair.

Reviews and reassessments

35. ...to be fully involved in the annual review procedure.
36. ...to complain if this is refused.
37. ...to request reassessment of their child if a change in circumstances occurs.
38. ...for their child to be the subject of a special annual review when aged fourteen which will include the production of a TRANSITION PLAN, the aim of which is to plan coherently for the young person's transition to adult life.
39. ...to request reassessment if they move to another area.
40. ...to have their child in receipt of full-time education up to the age of nineteen years.

General Advice

1. In all your contacts with your LEA or other organisation/ body/etc., keep carefully all letters you receive, make a copy of any letter you send out, note the date of *receipt* of any letter (as well as the date *on* the letter), keep a note of any telephone calls you make or receive.
Always note the name of any person to whom you speak, as well as their title, telephone number, extension number, etc., what was said on either side, etc.
If anything of importance is ever said to you in interview or

over the telephone, request that it be confirmed in writing within the near future.

2.   When writing to the LEA, particularly if protesting about or appealing against a decision, be as *factual* as possible and *not emotional.* State your case as plainly and simply as possible in the first instance and then add your reasons for thinking what you do. Give as many *facts* and as much *evidence* as possible to back up your case.

Try to be *positive* rather than negative and critical in what you write. State your case from your child's point of view rather than your own or that of another person. Prepare what you want to put across in rough first and check it in case there are any flaws or contradictions which need to be amended. (Getting a friend to go over what you have prepared could be very useful in this matter). At all times when writing, *concentrate on your child* and not on anyone or anything else.

For the sake of completeness the next chapter covers issues not so far dealt with but which are often encountered by a parent quite early on in the process of trying to learn about dyslexia.

Chapter 13: Other Issues/ Questions

The subject of dyslexia gives rise to many arguments between individuals and groups. A parent attempting to learn what he or she can about dyslexia is bound to run up against these debates sooner or later and before long could be in a position where it is necessary to 'take sides'. Parents will disagree with LEAs, LEAs will disagree with bodies such as the British Dyslexia Association (BDA) and Dyslexia Institute (DI), one psychologist will disagree with another and the medical world is likely to be in dispute with the field of education.

There are many matters which give rise to arguments but there are three in particular that cause more disagreement than most, these being:

*   Does dyslexia exist?
*   Is dyslexia more a medical or an educational matter?
*   Should difficulties with reading, spelling, writing etc. be called dyslexia or is specific learning difficulties (SpLDs) more accurate?

The professionals disagree also over other matters such as whether dyslexia can be diagnosed accurately, whether it is useful to talk about a child's potential in relation to dyslexia, whether differences between children are basically those of kind (qualitative) or merely degree (quantitative), and how accurate it is to claim that there are different types of dyslexia. However, the three singled out above get much more publicity than others and so we shall concentrate on them in this chapter.

1. Does Dyslexia Exist?

The existence of dyslexia is not accepted by every worker in the field of literacy difficulties. Many dedicated and highly respected psychologists and educationists, most of whom are based at universities and constantly involved in research, argue against the existence of such a phenomenon as dyslexia.

The attitude generally adopted is that those children referred to as dyslexic are not a separate group from other children who have reading difficulties caused by their being generally slow. They argue that dyslexic children are part of the whole group of children with reading difficulties and blend into one another in a gradual manner as part of a continuum. In other words, dyslexic children are not different *in kind* from other poor readers but only *in degree*. They will agree that there are *quantitative* differences, but not *qualitative* ones.

Because of the nature of the difficulties shown by the children we are concerned with, it is easy to understand why some workers should adopt this stance. In 1972 the Advisory Committee on Handicapped Children, which produced the Tizard Report, accepted that some children did experience severe and often long-lasting difficulties in learning to read, but found that there was no evidence to show that a collection of symptoms (i.e. a syndrome) of developmental dyslexia existed. However, the precise pattern of abilities which characterised the children considered to have a specific reading difficulty of any sort remained obscure. The Advisory Committee could *not* specify any procedure that could be used to identify such children.

More than 20 years have passed since then but the debate continues. In 1979–80 education and medical bodies (The Schools Council, the CSE Board, The GCE Board and The British Medical Association) were unable to formulate a working definition of the term dyslexia. In 1981 the Under-Secretary of State referred to dyslexia as a condition 'which is difficult to define' and also said that 'certain educationalists presume that it does not exist'. He also said, 'There is much stale argument over what is or is not dyslexia'.

In 1983 a government circular stated, 'Many educational and child psychologists had, and still have, serious reservations concerning the validity of the concept of dyslexia'.

At the present time some psychologists are willing to use the term dyslexia in a descriptive manner only. Others refuse to use the term at all as they consider the evidence on which the claim for the existence of dyslexia is based to be insufficient. The concept of dyslexia has come in for some very strong comments from some quarters. The late Professor Meredith of Leeds University referred to it as 'the unidentified flying object of psychology' and other critics have described it as a syndrome shown by the children of middle-class parents. However, most workers with objections to the concept of dyslexia express their reservations in a context of soundly based professional reasons.

The term 'dyslexia' is criticised because of the lack of an agreed working definition as well as there being no universally agreed means of alleviating the condition. The arbitrary nature of the dividing line between children considered to have some specific type of reading difficulty and those outside tends to be a matter of controversy. In our present state of knowledge, which is rather limited, we still do not know:

- the cause(s) of dyslexia;
- the exact signs or characteristics by which we can be sure that it is present in a child;
- how to identify it in every case;
- how to predict the manner in which it will develop within any particular child;
- exactly how to counteract its effects.

For a condition to exist in medicine or psychology one or more of these five characteristics should be present, otherwise we are on rather shaky ground. On the other hand, many conditions in the past were known to exist before they could be described so precisely. We now turn to the second main bone of contention.

2. Is Dyslexia a Medical or an Educational Matter?

The fact that two different professions are presently in dispute as to who is, so to speak, the rightful 'owner' of dyslexia is due to reasons which go back to the very origins of the discovery and description of dyslexia.

Because dyslexia relates to reading and reading-associated skills it is not surprising that it did not become properly detected or reported on by any professional person until education became more widespread and it was quite commonplace for ordinary people to be able to read and write.

It was not until 1877 that the loss of an adult's ability to read was professionally reported by a German physician, Kussmaul. However, as a point of interest it needs to be pointed out that the condition had almost certainly been encountered and remarked upon by others. For instance, the classic reforming novelist Charles Dickens in *Bleak House*, which was published in 1852, describes the character of Mr Krook, a ship's chandler, who is almost certainly dyslexic. He knows all the letters of the alphabet and can copy words from memory but cannot read them, despite having tried for the previous 25 years. He pastes up alphabets in the back room of his shop and is described as ' grubbing away at teaching himself to read and write, without getting on a bit'. He spells out words from papers which he has, 'chalking them over the table and the shop wall and asking people what this is and what this is...'. Another character says of Krook: 'Read! He'll never read. He can make all the letters separately and he knows most of them separately when he see them; he has got that much under me; but he can't put them together....'

It is quite probable that this description, published 25 years before Kussmaul described alexia (which he called 'word blindness'), is not the earliest one available.

The subject of dyslexia was virtually the exclusive property of the medical profession for the next 50 years or so, as Table 13.1 shows. The table lists the earliest historic milestones in the development of our knowledge about dyslexia.

Table 13.1: Milestones in knowledge about dyslexia					
Date	Name	Profession	Occupation	Term used	Had studied
1877	Kussmaul	Medicine	Physician	Word blindness	Adults
1887	Berlin	Medicine	Professor	Dyslexia	Adults
1895	Hinshelwood	Medicine	Eye surgeon	Word blindness	Adults
1896	Kerr	Medicine	Medical Officer of Health	Congenital word blindness	Children
1896	Pringle-Morgan	Medicine	General Practitioner	Congenital word blindness	Children
1925	Orton	Medicine	Psychiatrist	Specific reading difficulties	Children

As the table shows, a dyslexic-type difficulty was first officially reported in 1877 but was then called 'word blindness'. The German physician Kussmaul was describing the condition he had found in an adult who had originally been able to read but had then lost the ability to do so. The term 'word blindness' is an inaccurate one but nevertheless has stuck in the public mind and entered everyday speech, becoming quite firmly linked with the condition and giving it a medical type of association.

The condition Kussmaul described would nowadays be called alexia or acquired dyslexia. The term *dyslexia* was not used for a further 10 years, until Professor Berlin used it to describe the acquired condition, again in an adult. The developmental condition, which is found in children, was not reported officially until 1896 and in that year two different people, by sheer coincidence, did so. Both Dr James Kerr (a Medical Officer of Health in Bradford) and Dr Pringle-Morgan (a General Practitioner from the south coast) described various children they had encountered with the condition. They each used the term congenital word blindness and by means of such a form of words were able to convey the point that it was a condition the children had possessed throughout their lives; it had *not* been acquired as in the cases of adults described by the earlier reports. The term 'congenital word blindness' used by these two doctors is today known as 'developmental dyslexia' (which in this book we call simply 'dyslexia') and Kerr and Pringle-Morgan are acknowledged to be the discoverers of dyslexia in children

The medical profession was the only one to describe or report on the condition for many decades, as the first educational psychologist in Great Britain was not appointed until 1913. (This was Cyril Burt – who was later knighted – appointed to the London County Council). Psychologists during this period (the late 19th and early 20th centuries) did a great deal of work designed to help children and their parents overcome difficulties related to literacy. Cyril Burt produced much work of this nature and similar interest has been shown by the majority of educational psychologists who followed him into the profession.

When it is appreciated that medical personnel place emphasis on disorder, disease and treatment but that psychologists place emphasis on learning processes and development it is understandable that contrasting interpretations are inevitable. In 1981 McDonald Critchley (a neurologist) wrote that 'I have always insisted that the diagnosis of specific developmental dyslexia is a *medical* responsibility'. But in the same year Whittaker (an educational psychologist) wrote; 'We do not have a medical condition called dyslexia, we have an *educational* problem about how to teach more effectively'. These two workers and their viewpoints sum up the issue in the debate very effectively

As a final comment we need to say that the British Medical Association has advised its members that dyslexia is not basically a medical problem. For the sake of balance it also needs to be said that neurologists disagree with this. We now turn to the third dispute we need to discuss.

3. Dyslexia Versus Specific Learning Difficulties (SpLD)

The debate centres on which of these two is the more appropriate term to use when referring to children who have reading or other literacy difficulties.

As will be appreciated, the whole study of dyslexia has been handicapped from the earliest days by the use of different terms to describe the type of reading difficulties we are concerned with. We know from Table 13.1 that 'word blindness' and dyslexia were used in the case of adults and 'congenital word blindness' and 'specific reading difficulties' were used to refer to children. With the passage of time the labels have multiplied, each new one being introduced in an attempt to clarify matters and produce general acceptance.

'Congenital word blindness' is unsuitable as the condition is not any kind of blindness. 'Strephosymbolia' which was also used by Orton (who is listed in the table) means the twisting of symbols. It is not suitable as the confusion of letters such as 'b' and 'd' or words such as 'saw' and 'was' is only part of the total picture. 'Developmental dyslexia' has much to recommend it as the word 'developmental' clearly indicates that children and not adults are involved.

The manner in which dyslexia, or dyslexic-type difficulties, have been defined by various organisations over the last quarter century or so gives insight into the confusion and arguments which exist today. We have discussed these at some length in Chapter 6 and analysed the essential elements of them, comparing one with another, although it has not been necessary to give each definition at length. Of the five different names used by the seven different bodies/organisations dealt with in Chapter 6 it has been found that, over the years, three have tended to drop out of use with only two

- dyslexia, and
- specific learning difficulties remaining.

However, these two survive in an atmosphere of strong dispute. A number of different attitudes have been expressed, each by its own group of supporters. These are:

- dyslexia and SpLDs are different;
- dyslexia and SpLDs are the same;
- dyslexia is one of a number of SpLDs;
- it does not matter whether they are the same or not.

Generally speaking, dyslexia is the term favoured by most workers in the medical field whereas specific learning difficulties tends to be used by those in education. There is also the general assumption that dyslexia is a part (or subset) of SpLDs. Over the years psychologists have come to accept that there could be a VARIETY of specific developmental dyslexias (which is abbreviated to 'dyslexia') and that these could all be included within specific learning difficulties (SpLDs) as these constitute a wide group of difficulties.

Many parents, teachers and psychologists are in agreement that such matters are irrelevant and that all energy ought to be invested in being able to identify the children concerned more effectively by accurate assessment methods, as well as being able to assist them by more effective teaching techniques.

We finish this chapter by answering a number of questions commonly asked by parents but not covered in Chapter 7.

Is dyslexia inherited?

For almost a century it has been known that any child with dyslexia is likely to have one or more close relatives who are dyslexic also; dyslexia runs in families. However, it was not known for certain whether this situation arose because dyslexia was capable of being inherited or rather because the dyslexic family members shared the same environment and it was something related to the environment which brought the dyslexia about.

Recent studies have concentrated on twins (both identical and non-identical types) or other family members. The results have shown that there is a genetic cause; dyslexia *can* be inherited. In fact this is a gross over-simplification of the situation. What is inherited is not dyslexia itself but aspects of phonological processing which, if

deficient, can produce difficulties in learning to read. Further work
has shown that deficits in phonological skills are themselves the result
of an inherited weakness in segmental language skills and so the situation can be summarised roughly as in Figure 13.1.

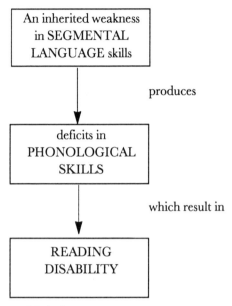

Figure 13.1 Heredity aspects of dyslexia

The exact means by which the dyslexia is inherited is not yet known
but there are several possible mechanisms. Every human being devel-
ops from a single egg which contains 23 pairs of thin threads called
chromosomes. One of each pair comes from the father and the other
from the mother. All of our chromosomes are set by the contents of this
first single cell. Each chromosome is made up of a string of small genes
and each gene carries the hereditary chemicals which distinguish our
characteristics – height, weight, skin pigmentation, eye colour, suscep-
tibility to disease etc. Each pair of chromosomes is different from all
other pairs. They have been numbered for identification purposes and
the genes strung out along them are in the process of being mapped
out in great detail. Deficits, weaknesses and mutations are passed on
from one generation to the next if one gene on one chromosome
becomes altered appropriately. One pair of genes determines the sex
of the individual and sometimes defects are passed on by these genes
and so become sex-linked characteristics.

It is possible that dyslexia is brought about by the combined influence of a number of genes but there is also evidence to suggest that it is caused by a single dominant gene. The exact situation is as yet far from clear-cut and work is still very much ongoing. Some research has produced evidence that chromosome 15 is linked to dyslexia but other studies have not confirmed this. There is also evidence for a linkage on chromosome 6 and this evidence has been gathered from at least two independent sources and was reported on in late 1994. (Interestingly, the point on chromosome 6 which has been identified is in the same region as the human leukocyte antigen complex and may explain an often-reported association between dyslexia and auto-immune disease.)

People working in the field of heredity/genetics have shown that there is as much as a 50% probability of a boy becoming dyslexic if his father is dyslexic. The chances drop to about 40% if it is his mother who is affected. There is a lower probability still of a girl developing dyslexia in similar circumstances.

However, to put the situation into its correct perspective it needs also to be stated that environmental factors play a substantial role in the word recognition skills of children with dyslexia. One of the most important environmental factors is reading experience. In other words, reading will improve more in a child the more that child is exposed to the printed word. This applies even to those children who have severe deficits in their phonological skills. Hence genetic influences may constrain the speed or ease of reading development but environmental factors – such as improved reading instruction and greater reading experience – may compensate for the constraints imposed.

Dyslexics can eventually achieve high levels of word recognition but still tend to remain deficient in phonological coding skills. Hence reading experience alone may not be sufficient and recent work has looked at matters such as the training of particular language skills in children who are at the pre-reading stage. Such training may reduce the likelihood of reading difficulties later on.

Why are more boys than girls dyslexic?

Dyslexic boys outnumber girls by a ratio of 3, 4 or even 5 to 1. One suggested reason is that dyslexia is a sex-linked phenomenon but it is also suggested that the cause is boys developing more slowly than girls.

Are there signs by which we can identify dyslexic children?

There are no 'hard' signs and the question of whether there are 'soft' signs is one surrounded by confusion. Complications at the time of birth can lead to some children having reading difficulties later in life but this does not apply in all cases. There is no single 'soft' sign associated with dyslexia and so searches have been made for a *group of signs*. Signs such as difficulty in sequencing, mirror writing, letter reversals, cross laterality and finger agnosia have been suggested. However, there is no general agreement about their significance as they are often present in efficient readers.

Are reading difficulties associated with speech problems or delayed speech?

There is a substantial amount of evidence confirming that some children with speech defects have dyslexia or retardation in reading.

Do hearing problems cause reading difficulties?

Yes, in all children affected irrespective of whether the difficulties are dyslexic or not.

Are dyslexic children likely to have behaviour problems?

It is quite possible that these will develop. The DFE makes specific mention of them in the *Code of Practice* (in Section 3:61). It talks about severe emotional and behavioural difficulties (indicated by withdrawn or disruptive behaviour) which are sometimes associated with specific learning difficulties. It also mentions an inability to concentrate and indicates that the child experiences considerable frustration or distress in relation to his or her learning difficulties.

Do dyslexic children have handwriting problems or do they produce mirror-writing?

Some dyslexic children demonstrate handwriting problems as do some non-dyslexics. The same applies to mirror-writing. The cause could be maturational lag or some kind of generalised response of some children beginning to learn to write. It could be that these children are paying attention only to a letter's shape and not its orientation, i.e. they could be learning a bad habit very efficiently. It is also possible that poor handwriting or reversals are caused by uncertainty and confusion about how to write down what they want to say.

Is dyslexia the result of a language deficiency?

Research suggests that it is various deficits in language which are at the root of reading problems – but the link is a tenuous one. A more reasonable explanation could be that the language difficulties are the *result* of a child's lack of reading progress. Also, many children who have no language deficits still find reading difficult.

We now move on to devote a few pages to names and addresses of useful organisations.

Chapter 14:
Useful Information

It goes without saying that it is hoped that every parent of a dyslexic child will meet with goodwill and cooperation from all concerned in the education system and that as a result their child will be identified early, assessed without delay, have their needs fully described and then met; that the LEA will lay on appropriate resources to an adequate degree, keep the child's progress under regular review and maintain the situation while the needs remain.

Even were this ideal situation actually to be borne out there is no doubt that the parent concerned would still benefit a great deal from knowledge about their rights, their child's rights, voluntary agencies, support groups etc.

In the case of a parent who encounters hostility, indifference, opposing viewpoints, lack of action, unwarranted delays etc., support is vital and one of the best forms is to provide the parent with the information they need to be able to muster support for their child so as to present his case as strongly as possible.

That is what this chapter is all about – to let parents know about useful publications, support agencies and organisations in general who are able to provide information, guidance and general help. They have been grouped under three main readings relating to Local Education Authorities (LEAs), independent organisations which exist in order to assist in any type of case of special educational needs and finally those concerned only with dyslexic children. As a preliminary you might find it useful to know the whereabouts of the

Department for Education which is responsible for the education system of England and Wales:

THE DEPARTMENT FOR EDUCATION
SANCTUARY BUILDINGS
GREAT SMITH STREET
WESTMINSTER
LONDON SW1P 3BT
(Telephone: 0171 925 5000)

Your Local Education Authority (LEA)

1.   Every *LEA* must produce a *booklet* of general information for parents and update it annually. You may have one free of charge on request. In it there should be set out the LEA's policy on children with special educational needs and a description of what resources it has to meet those needs.

2.   Every LEA *school* must produce a *booklet* describing the school's philosophy, policy on relevant matters and details relating to special educational needs. You should be able to obtain a copy for the school your child attends. If a change of school is suggested as a means of assisting with his dyslexia you should be able to obtain a copy of the booklet relating to the proposed school. Again, these booklets are to be updated annually.

Independent Bodies (Special Needs in General)

3.   If you have been involved in an appeal held in connection with the assessment of your child's special educational needs and you feel that the behaviour of the Appeal Committee was unfair then you can complain to:

COUNCIL ON TRIBUNALS
ST DUNSTAN'S HOUSE
FETTER LANE
LONDON
EC4R 1BT
(Telephone: 0171 404 4954)

who may arrange a hearing.

4.   If you are unhappy about the manner in which your LEA has dealt with your child's special educational needs you may

appeal beyond it to the Secretary of State and have your case heard at a Special Educational Needs Tribunal. You can write to him or her at the Department for Education. Your local Citizens Advice Bureau or any of a number of other organisations can help you with this.

5.   You may find that being a member of a group will be of assistance to you. There may be a local group of CASE in your area. More information can be obtained from:

CAMPAIGN FOR THE ADVANCEMENT OF STATE EDUCATION (CASE)
25 LEYBORNE PARK
KEW GARDENS
RICHMOND
SURREY
TW0 3HB

6.   Information and advice about all aspects of the State Education service is offered by the ADVISORY CENTRE FOR EDUCATION (ACE) whose address is:

1B ABERDEEN STUDIOS
22–24 HIGHBURY GROVE
LONDON
N5 2EA
(Telephone: 0171 354 8321)

7.   ACE publishes the ACE Special Education Handbook which you will probably find very useful and informative and the telephone HELPLINE is open on weekdays from 2–5 pm.

8.   The CSIE aims to ensure that LEAs, individual schools, parents and others establish effective and stable integration schemes for children with special needs.

CENTRE FOR STUDIES ON INTEGRATION IN EDUCATION (CSIE)
4TH FLOOR
415 EDGWARE ROAD
LONDON
NW2 6NB
(Telephone 0181 452 8642)

9.   Free information and an advice service by TELEPHONE
      relating to those laws and policies which affect children and
      young people in England and Wales is provided by:

      THE CHILDREN'S LEGAL CENTRE
      20 COMPTON TERRACE
      LONDON
      N1 2UN
      (Telephone: 0171 359 6251/9392)

10.   An independent panel of special education experts is also
      available at this address and will help parents who want a
      second opinion.

11.   A free information service and a range of free publications is
      available from:

      THE VOLUNTARY COUNCIL FOR HANDICAPPED
      CHILDREN
      8 WAKLEY STREET
      LONDON
      EC1V 7QE
      (Telephone: 0171 843 6000)

12.   You may at some time need to consult an ombudsman, the
      address of whom is:

      LOCAL GOVERNMENT OMBUDSMAN
      21 QUEEN ANNE'S GATE
      LONDON
      SW1H 9BU
      (Telephone: 0171 222 5622)

Independent Bodies (concerned with Dyslexia)

13.   Much of the work in relation to children with dyslexia who live
      in the British Isles is carried out by the British Dyslexia Associ-
      ation and the Dyslexia Institute, with other bodies and organ-
      isations providing additional and much valued contributions.
      Taking them in order, we have:

BRITISH DYSLEXIA ASSOCIATION
98 LONDON ROAD
READING
BERKSHIRE
RG1 5AU
(Telephone: 01734 668271)

The BDA provides advice and information on resources, work-shops, clubs, LEA initiatives and regional networks. A magazine *Contact* is published twice a year and other literature is also available. (You will be able to find out from the BDA whether there is a branch near to you).

14.   You may also want to contact:

THE BDA COMPUTER RESOURCE CENTRE
DEPARTMENT OF PSYCHOLOGY
UNIVERSITY OF HULL
HULL
HU6 7RX
(Telephone: 01482 465388)

which contains a wide range of software which learners with dyslexia have found to be of value. Teachers or parents can visit the centre (by appointment) or write/phone in with any queries.

15.   The Dyslexia Institute has a number of centres throughout the UK to provide educational and psychological assessment of children and adults, special tuition, teacher training and information.

THE DYSLEXIA INSTITUTE
133 GRESHAM ROAD
STAINES
MIDDLESEX
TW18 2AJ
(Telephone: 01784 463851)

16.   The National Federation of ACCESS centres is a nationwide group of Further Education (FE) establishments which assess adult students and recommend suitable software and aids.

They undertake assessment for the Open University and for LEAs. Recently they have begun to help students with specific learning difficulties.

NATIONAL FEDERATION OF ACCESS CENTRES
HEREWARD COLLEGE OF FURTHER EDUCATION
BRAMSTON CRESCENT
TILE HILL LANE
COVENTRY
CV4 9SW
(Telephone: 01203 461231)

17.   PATOSS is the Professional Association of Teachers of Students with Specific Learning Difficulties. It is a recently formed professional body representing those who hold the nationally recognised RSA Diploma in Specific Learning Difficulties. Its aim is to raise the level of debate at national level as well as to influence decision makers.

PATOSS
c/o HILARY GREEN
SUNNYBANK
CHURCHILL
OX7 6NW
(Telephone: 01608 658657)

18.   The National Council for Educational Technology was set up by the DES (now DFE) in April 1988 to promote the use of new technologies in education. There is a Special Needs action which undertakes projects in the special needs area and dyslexia is included in this. It produces information sheets and suggestions for ways of working.

NCET
SIR WILLIAM LYONS ROAD
UNIVERSITY OF WARWICK SCIENCE PARK
COVENTRY
CV4 7EZ
(Telephone: 01203 416994)

19.   The Helen Arkell Dyslexia Centre arranges consultancies, assessments by educational psychologists, teachers and speech therapists,

provides tuition, speech and language therapy, counselling and various types of training, e.g. keyboarding skills etc.

THE HELEN ARKELL DYSLEXIA CENTRE
FRENSHAM
FARNHAM
SURREY
GU10 3DW
(Telephone: 01252 792400)

Finally, if you live outside England and Wales, you might like to know that there is both a Scottish and an Irish Dyslexia Association. In the following chapter, which is the last of the book, a brief history of dyslexia is set out.

Chapter 15:
A Brief History of Dyslexia

What follows below and on the next pages is a summary of the key events in the story of how dyslexia came to be recognised, described and to grow in the awareness of people worldwide until it has achieved the status it enjoys today. Most details given are in relation to Britain but some developments in other parts of the world are also included.

Date	Britain	Elsewhere
	Before the year 1500 people considered that thoughts and feelings originated in the heart.	
1500	After 1500 it slowly became realised that the *brain* was the organ involved.	
1800	About 1800 scientists realised that the faculty of language was located within the cerebral hemispheres and that loss of speech was due to a malfunction of the brain and not the tongue.	
1861	The connection was established between the frontal lobes of the brain and the impairment of speech.	
1865		Broca concluded that speech control was located in the left half of the brain only and not both sides.
		• Later it was realised that this does not apply to all people but is true in the case of the great majority.
		• The name *aphasia* was applied to those cases of people who had lost the power of speech.
		• Eventually it was realised that a

Date	Britain	Elsewhere
		number of aphasias existed – some in which reading and writing was affected as well as speech, others in which reading and writing were seriously affected but speech only to a lesser extent. This latter group were then described as 'word blind' but today would be called 'alexic'.
1870	The Forster Education Act granted an elementary level of education to all children. Large numbers of children could be observed by teachers and others over a lengthy period of time. Reading difficulties came to be studied more widely.	
1877		Kussmaul described alexia which he called 'word blindness'.
1879		Wundt in Leipzig set up the first psychology laboratory and thereby instituted the modern scientific approach to the subject.
1887		Professor Berlin first used the word DYSLEXIA to describe ALEXIA.
1896	Kerr and Pringle-Morgan described DYSLEXIA in children, calling it 'congenital word blindness'.	
Late 19th century	Throughout this period the early psychologists pioneered psychologically-based methods of helping children with reading difficulties.	
1913	First educational psychologist in the British Isles (Cyril Burt – later knighted for his service to education) appointed by the London County Council.	

Date	Britain	Elsewhere
1920s onwards	Much work carried out in relation to reading difficulties by Burt and Schonnell.	
1920s		(USA) Orton noted that an immensely high proportion of children with specific reading disability were producing mirror-writing and had orientation difficulties.
1938		(DENMARK) Edith Norrie founded the first organisation in the world devoted to diagnosing and teaching dyslexics, THE WORD BLIND INSTITUTE, Copenhagen.
1949		(USA) The Orton Society was founded but later was called the Orton Dyslexia Society. It produced *The Bulletin of the Orton Society* which was later renamed *Annals of Dyslexia*.
1950s (early)	St Bartholomew's Hospital (London) became involved in the diagnosis and treatment of dyslexic children. Other hospitals also showed an interest and carried out work.	(SOUTH AFRICA) Rebecca Oistrowick started work and was one of the pioneers who used multi-sensory methods.
1960	Maisie Holt, a psychologist, started teaching dyslexic children at the instigation of Dr Franklin White, a paediatrician, who afterwards became Chairman of the Invalid Children's Aid Association (ICAA). A clinic was set up which gave free help to large numbers of children and adults, paid for by the NHS.	

Date	*Britain*	*Elsewhere*
	The Hornsby Centre in Wandsworth and the Hornsby School were offshoots of this.	
1963	The ICAA established the Word Blind Centre for Dyslexic Children in London. (It closed in 1972 having been intended only as a short-term measure.) However, the establishment of the Centre was probably the point at which dyslexia started to become known to the public at large and generated a great deal of interest.	
1960s (mid)	The Dyslexia Unit was set up at the University College of North Wales, Bangor by Professor T. Miles in order to undertake assessments and carry out research.	
1965 (to 1972)	Eight voluntary dyslexia associations were started.	
1967		(AUSTRALIA) SPELD (which stands for *Specific Learning Diffi*culties was set up in New South Wales. The movement grew, spreading throughout Australia, Tasmania and New Zealand.
1970	The Chronically Sick and Disabled Persons Act passed. The word 'dyslexia' was first mentioned by the legal system.	
1971	The Helen Arkell Dyslexia Centre was set up. (It is now located at Frensham, Surrey).	
1972	1. The Dyslexia Institute was set up by the North Surrey Dyslexia Association. It now has many institutes,	

Date	*Britain*	*Elsewhere*
	outposts and schools throughout England, Scotland and Guernsey. 2. The British Dyslexia Association (BDA) was founded by Marion Welchman. It is the national organisation and the parent body to which local associations are affiliated. At present there are in excess of 70 of these. The BDA is based in Reading. 3. The Tizard Report was published. It recommended the use of the term 'specific reading difficulties'.	
1975	*Alpha to Omega* published.	
1977	The BDA established formal links with the DES (now DFE).	
1978	The Warnock Report *Special Educational Needs* published.	
1980	The British Medical Association advised its members that dyslexia is not a medical problem.	
1981	1. Education Act passed. It became possible for a dyslexic child to have his or her special educational needs protected by the issuing of a formal 'Statement of Special Educational Needs'. 2. Tansley and Panckhurst published *Children with Specific Learning Difficulties*.	
1982	1. The Watford Dyslexia Unit was set up by Violet Brand. 2. The City of London Dyslexia Institute training unit was opened.	
1983	The 1981 Education Act was	

Date	Britain	Elsewhere
	enacted as from 1 April.	
1987		The European Dyslexia Association (EDA) was formed.
1988		The European Dyslexia Association was given the Belgian Royal Assent.
1989	The British Dyslexia Association organised the first international conference on dyslexia which was very successful.	
1988/ 89	A survey of 882 educational psychologists in relation to specific learning difficulties/dyslexia was organised by Professor Pumfrey and Ms Reason (Sen Ed Psych) based at the School of Education, Manchester University.	
1991	The BDA organised the second international conference on dyslexia.	
1992	Dyslexia Institute Week (2–8 March) organised by the Dyslexia Institute.	
1993	Education Act 1993	
1994		1. 26–27 March in Brussels representatives from all the European Union countries met for the very first time to discuss specialist teaching for dyslexia.
	2. The DFE published the Code of Practice on the Identification of Special Needs in which clear guidelines are given to LEAs and governing bodies of all main tained schools about their responsibilities to children with specific learning difficulties (for example dyslexia). The Code came into effect on 1 September 1994.	
1995	1. The Booksellers Association (the trade association representing	

the interests of all book retailers)
adopts the British Dyslexia
Association for 1995 (the Book-
sellers Association's Centenary year).
2.The Joint Council for the GCSE's
special arrangements and special
considerations, which includes
children with specific learning
difficulties, became effective
in and from summer 1995.
3.Schools must publish information
on their SEN policies by 1st August 1995.

Appendix

The definitions used in Chapter 6 are given here in full:

(A) *Dyslexia*: 'A disorder in children who, despite conventional class-room experience, fail to attain the language skills of reading, writing and spelling commensurate with their intellectual abilities' (World Federation of Neurology, 1968).

(B) *Dyslexia*: 'We define dyslexia as a specific difficulty in learning, constitutional in origin, in one or more of reading, spelling and written language which may be accompanied by difficulty in number work. It is particularly related to mastering and using written language (alphabetic, numerical and musical notation) although often affecting oral language to some degree' (British Dyslexia Association, 1989).

(C) *Specific developmental dyslexia*: 'A disorder manifested by difficulty in learning to read despite conventional instruction, adequate intelligence, and socio-cultural opportunity. It depends on fundamental cognitive disabilities which are frequently of constitutional origin' (World Federation of Neurology, 1968).

(D) *Specific reading retardation*: '... an attainment on either reading accuracy or reading comprehension which was 28 months or more below the level predicted on the basis of each child's age and short WISC IQ' (Rutter, Tizard and Whitmore, 1970).

(E) *Specific learning difficulties*: 'Children with specific learning difficulties are those who in the absence of sensory defect or overt organic damage, have an intractable learning problem in one or more of reading, writing, spelling and mathematics, and who do not respond to normal teaching. For these children, early identification, sensitive encouragement and specific remedial arrangements are necessary' (Tansley and Panckhurst, 1981).

(F) *Specific learning difficulties*: These 'are defined as organising or learning deficiencies which restrict the student's competencies in information processing, in motor skills and working memory, so causing limitations in some or all of the skills of speech, reading, writing, essay writing, numeracy and behaviour' (Dyslexia Institute, 1989).

(G) *Specific reading difficulties*: A descriptive term used to indicate the problems of the relatively small proportion of pupils 'whose reading (and perhaps writing, spelling and number) abilities are significantly below the standards which their abilities in other spheres would lead one to expect'. (DES, 1972).

Glossary

ACE Advisory Centre for Education.

ACID (test) An expression used in relation to the results obtained from a dyslexic child when given the WISC. Low scores on the Arithmetic, Coding, Information and Digit span sub-tests are claimed by some researchers to result often, and the four initials of these sub-tests when combined together produce ACID.

acquired dyslexia Also known as alexia, this is one of the two main types of dyslexia and is the form found in adults. It refers to the loss of the ability to read by a person who was previously able to do so.

acute dyslexia A misleading term, as dyslexia cannot be acute in the medical sense of 'coming sharply to a crisis'. The term was used in the Chronically Sick and Disabled Persons Act of 1970 and its use caused some confusion. It is presumed that 'acute' means 'severe'.

agnosia The inability to recognise familiar sounds, images, etc. There are various forms such as visual agnosia, auditory agnosia and tactile agnosia. (See also finger agnosia.)

AHA Area Health Authority.

alexia Also known as acquired dyslexia, this is one of the two main types of dyslexia and is the form in adults. A person with alexia has lost the ability to read, usually as a result of head injury, brain tumour or the effect of drugs etc.

aphasia Loss of, or impairment to, the ability to use language because of damage to the brain. Expressive aphasia is the inability to produce a required word even though the word is known to the person affected. Receptive aphasia involves the understanding of speech. There are other aphasias. Any person affected is described as aphasic.

aqueous humour The clear, watery liquid which fills the front part of the eye between the cornea and the lens.

ARROW Aural–Read–Response–Oral–Written

attentional dyslexia A sub-type of alexia (acquired dyslexia) claimed to exist by at least one researcher.

auditory dyslexia A sub-type of developmental dyslexia such that the child cannot associate the printed image of the word with the sound the word makes. Such children respond best to a whole-word 'look-and-say' approach during the initial stages of reading as they are unable to break down a word into the smaller sounds (phonemes) which compose the word.

backward reader One who reads less well than most other children at the same age due to having a lower basic ability (intelligence level) and hence being unable to read any better (compare with *Retarded reader*).

BDA British Dyslexia Association.

CA Chronological age.

CAL Computer-assisted learning.

capital (letter) The large form of a letter of the alphabet used at the start of proper names and to begin a sentence. Also known as *upper-case* (derived from the printing trade). (Compare with *small letter*.)

CASE Campaign for the Advancement of State Education.

cerebral cortex The grey surface of the brain, a layer only 3mm thick and composed of more than one million million nerve cells, each with connections to many thousands of others. Underneath the cerebral cortex is the brain's white matter.

cerebral hemisphere One half of the brain, there being a left and a right cerebral hemisphere separated by the deep longitudinal fissure which runs from front to back.

Certificate of Secondary Education (CSE) An examination designed to be taken by school leavers as an alternative to GCE 'O' Level. It was introduced in 1965 but was discontinued after 1987, being replaced by the GCSE.

chronological age A person's age in the everyday meaning of the word – the amount of time that has elapsed since he or she was born. Often abbreviated to CA. A child can be described in terms of other ages also, e.g. developmental age, reading age, mental age.

Cloze procedure A method designed to measure how readable a book is. A child attempts to read a passage from which some words have been removed. How easily he is able to give the words which should occupy the blank spaces is taken as a measure of the passage's readability.

CMO Clinical Medical Officer. Formerly known as SMO (School Medical Officer) or, simply, School Doctor.

cones Highly specialised cells in the retina (the light-sensitive layer at the back of the eyeball). The cones respond to different colours and there are six million of them in each eye. They work in close association with the *rods*.

congenital Literally this means 'appearing with birth' but has unfortunately become confused in the minds of many people with 'hereditary' and this is incorrect. Anything hereditary is handed on from parent to child whereas something congenital (e.g. a disease) can arise after conception but before birth. Hereditary diseases are congenital but congenital diseases are not necessarily hereditary.

congenital dyslexia One of a number of terms used to describe developmental dyslexia.

congenital word blindness One of the many terms used to described developmental dyslexia. It was first used by Kerr (a Medical Office of Health) and Pringle-Morgan (a General Practitioner) in 1896.

conjunctiva The thin transparent sheet of membrane which covers the front of the eye.

control group/controls A group of individuals that matches, as closely as possible, another group that is being experimented on in some way. As the controls are treated the same way in all respects *EXCEPT* any relating to the experiment, any differences that result in the second group must be as a result of the experimental treatment they have been given. A control group is a reference.

cornea A clear, transparent layer at the front of the eyeball, which is the window of the eye. The thin *conjunctiva* is on the outside surface and the inside surface is in contrast with the *aqueous humour*. Light rays pass through it, permitting us to see.

corpus callosum A large bundle of fibres in the brain which lies immediately below the longitudinal fissure. It bridges the two halves of the brain (cerebral hemispheres) and so allows 'signals' to pass from one half to the other.

correlation The manner in which two sets of measures vary together, e.g. shops sell more ice-cream when the weather is hot, taller people buy larger shoes, young children tend to weigh little and older children much more. Correlation can be measured mathematically and correlations can vary between very positive to very negative. (The three examples given are all positive as an increase in one leads to an increase in the other.)

cross-lateral A description of a person who prefers to use different sides of his body for different purposes, e.g. the right eye for sighting something but the left hand for throwing a ball.

CSE Certificate of Secondary Education.

CSIE Centre for Studies on Integration in Education.

DATAPAC Daily Teaching and Assessment (Primary Aged Children).

deep dyslexia A sub-type of alexia. People who have deep dyslexia cannot connect a word they see in print with the sound of the word. Familiar words are read more easily than unfamiliar ones and abstract words are particularly difficult for them. Meaningful substitutions are made for difficult words.

DES Department of Education and Science (now known as the Department for Education – DFE).

DFE Department for Education.

developmental aphasia Term used in the literature to describe dyslexia (according to Miles).

developmental dyslexia The type of dyslexia found in children and called by many names. It is different from *acquired dyslexia* which occurs in adults.

DI Dyslexia Institute.

direct dyslexia Also called '*hyperlexia*' and one of the sub-types of *acquired dyslexia* which is found in adults. Individuals are able to read quite accurately but the meaning of what they have read is understood quite poorly. Whilst phonological and whole-word strategies are competent their semantic analysis skills are deficient.

discrepancy A difference or inconsistency.

dominance (1) The fact that one half of the brain exercises more power over the body than does the other. *This is cerebral dominance.* (2) The preferred use of one side of the body. If right eye, right hand and right leg are preferred by a person (s)he is *right-side dominant* and if the others are preferred (s)he is *left-side dominant.* One who uses different sides of the body for different tasks (e.g. right hand but left eye) is *cross-dominant.* If a person uses both the left and the right of a pair of limbs with equal ease (as does someone ambidextrous) then (s)he is described as having *mixed dominance*. (Dominance in this second sense is similar to laterality).

dominant hemisphere (i) The half of the brain on the opposite side of the body to the preferred hand. The left hemisphere is the dominant one for most people. (ii) In relation to a *particular* activity or function (such as language), the half of the brain which controls it. In the case of language the left hemisphere controls 90% of right-handed people but only 30% of left-handed people.

DORRS Development of Reading and Related Skills with Pupils of Secondary Age.

dyseidetic dyslexia A sub-group of dyslexic children (according to Boder). The word is of Greek origin and indicates a difficulty with images or what is being looked at. A dyseidetic child is described as one who has difficulties with visuo-spatial aspects. More simply, there is difficulty experienced in the ability to perceive letters and whole words as belonging together. See *dysphonetic dyslexia* and *mixed (dyseidetic/dysphonetic) dyslexia.*.

dyslexia *In the case of children* dyslexia is a difficulty in learning to read which is often associated with other difficulties (such as spelling and writing) and for which there is no obvious explanation such as low intelligence, visual defects, lack of adequate and consistent schooling etc.

There are two forms of dyslexia, the other one relating to adults who had previously been able to read and the lost their ability to do so (alexia). Both forms have been given a variety of names in the century and more which has elapsed since the condition was first described. Both types have been described as being composed of sub-groupings and many names describing these sub-groups have been given. Dyslexia in children is a highly controversial topic with every aspect of the subject, even its very existence, being strongly debated. *Specific learning difficulties* is the name preferred by many.

dysphonetic dyslexia A sub-group of dyslexic children (according to Boder). The word is of Greek origin and indicates a difficulty with sounds. A dysphonetic child is described as having difficulties with sound-symbol relations. More simply, the child is unable to look at the printed word, analyse it into its basic sounds and then synthesise (or blend) them together in order to say the word (correctly). See *dyseidetic dyslexia* and *mixed (dyseidetic/dysphonetic) dyslexia*.

educational psychologist (EP) A person who has (1) a first degree in psychology (usually an Honours) (2) a postgraduate qualification in educational psychology (usually a Masters degree) (3) a teaching qualification (4) a minimum of two years' teaching experience. EPs are usually employed by Local Education Authorities (LEAs) although some work for other bodies and yet more are in private practice. EPs are responsible for carrying out assessments on children suspected of having special educational needs and for giving appropriate advice as to how those needs would be best met. Other types of work are also undertaken by them in their involvement with children, parents and teachers.

EEG Electroencephalogram.

electroencephalogram A record of the electrical activity of the brain. Different types of brain activity produce regular wave patterns (rhythms) and these are called alpha, beta, delta, theta. The patient's scalp is wired to an electroencephalograph machine which records the patterns on a continuous sheet of paper. Irregular patterns can be a clue to brain damage, epilepsy etc. and up to 16 'channels' may be recorded.

EP Educational psychologist.

EPS Educational Psychology Service.

EWO Education Welfare Officer.

eye dominance A term used to describe the fact that most people have one eye which they prefer over the other when sighting (e.g. in using a telescope). About two-thirds of the population prefer to use their right eye. Several theories suggest that eye dominance is important in relation to dyslexia.

eye tracking The movement of the eye when scanning something. In reading most people 'track' or follow the line of print from left to right. There are reports of a high incidence of tracking from right to left among dyslexic people which, if accurate, could account for some reading difficulties.

factor An influence or force. Something which affects the outcome of an event. The length of a rectangle is one factor in deciding its area. Soil richness is a factor involved in how high a tree will grow.

filter A sheet of material, usually in the form of spectacle lenses or a page overlay which is tinted and removes certain light wavelengths.

finger agnosia The inability of a person to know, when blindfolded, how many of his fingers have been touched. (At one time this was employed by Professor Miles as part of a battery of tests aimed at detecting dyslexic children but eventually he did not feel justified in continuing with it.)

fissure A deep cleft or separation in the surface of the brain, a shallow cleft being termed a *sulcus*.

flash card A large card on which a word is printed and employed by teachers in the teaching of reading. The flash card is shown to the class for a very brief period of time to increase the speed at which they can recognise the word. Flash cards complement the whole-word 'look-and-say' method and are often used in remedial work.

frontal lobe The lobe on each cerebral hemisphere which lies to the front of the brain and is separated from the lobes behind by the central fissure.

GCE General Certificate of Education.

GCSE General Certificate of Secondary Education.

General Certificate of Education (GCE) The 'O' level and 'A' level examination taken up until 1987 and then replaced by the GCSE.

General Certificate of Secondary Education (GCSE) In 1988 the GCSE examination replaced the GCE and the CSE 'O' level examinations.

graphemic processor dyslexia Another name for visual processor dyslexia.

grey matter The name given to the thin outer layer (cerebral cortex) of the brain. Underneath is the white matter. In the spine the grey and white matters are reversed with the grey matter being on the inside.

gyrus A ridge of the brain's surface.

'hard' signs (of brain damage) Usually the actual injury, wound or scar.

homograph A word which is *spelled* the same as another word but happens to be pronounced differently as it has a different meaning, e.g. 'I can hear the *wind* in the trees' *but* 'Now I will *wind* the clock' (see also *homonym* and *homophone*).

homonym A word which has at least two completely different senses, e.g. 1. BANK – (i) a building (ii) a piece of land; 2. POLE – (i) a piece of wood (ii) a native of Poland (iii) an old-fashioned measure of length (see also *homophone* and *homograph*).

homophone A word which sounds the same as another word of different meaning, e.g. 1. sale – sail, 2. horse – hoarse, 3. saw – sore – soar (see also *homonym* and *homograph*).

hyperlexia See *direct dyslexia*.

hypothesis A supposition made as a starting point for an investigation.

ICAA Invalid Children's Aid Association.

incidence The frequency with which an event occurs. The incidence of cystic fibrosis is 1 in every 2000–2500. The incidence of dyslexia has varied a great deal between one claim and another but 4 in 100 appears to be the most commonly agreed figure.

inorganic books Traditional reading books which are designed to teaching reading in a formal manner. There is much repetition and often a rather artificial style of language. They are to be contrasted with *organic books.*

International Phonetic Alphabet (IPA) An alphabet produced by the International Phonetic Association to provide symbols for the sounds of any language. It has been revised on a number of occasions since the first version, the latest being in 1989. A total of 98 symbols are employed, 44 of which apply to ordinary English (Received Pronunciation).

IPA 1. International Phonetic Alphabet. 2. International Phonetic Association.

IQ Intelligence quotient.

ITA Initial Teaching Alphabet.

kinaesthetic The kinaesthetic sense, or kinaesthesis, is that which enables us to appreciate the positions and movements of our limbs. It depends on specialised receptor cells in muscles, tendons and joints.

lateral geniculate nucleus There is a lateral geniculate nucleus in each cerebral hemisphere. They are involved with the visual process and are an important part of the visual pathway. The vision 'signals' from the two eyes are passed to the lateral geniculate nucleus and inside are transferred to the nerves which pass back through the optic radiations to the rear of the brain.

laterality The preference for using the right or left side of the body. The development of laterality is of assistance to the child in acquiring a full sense of bodily awareness and general coordination. See *dominance.*

LEA Local Education Authority

learning difficulty A child has a learning difficulty if he requires something additional to, or different from, the majority of other children of the same age in order to pursue the normal school curriculum within his LEA. Note that this is a different meaning from that of everyday usage. (A child in a wheelchair is considered to have a learning difficulty by this description yet that child could be a high achiever and display no difficulties in the ordinary learning process.)

legasthenia One of the many terms for dyslexia used in the past.

lens (i) The part of the eye which focuses the incoming light rays on to the retina at the rear (ii) Specially shaped pieces of glass or plastic in spectacles in order to assist with vision defects.

lexical system That which relates to the words of a language.

Look-and-Say (method of teaching reading) Also called the whole-word method, the child is encouraged to recognise a word (or group of words) by shape when this method is used. It is most commonly employed in the early stages of reading in order to build up the child's sight vocabulary and is rarely used entirely on its own. It is to be contrasted with the *phonic* method.

lower case (letter) The 'small' form of the letters of the alphabet, as opposed to the 'capitals'. (The term 'lower case' is one associated with the printing trade).

'L' type dyslexia A sub-group of dyslexic children (as claimed by Bakker) and one of two, the other being 'P' type. An 'L' type of dyslexic child is described as reading in a hurried fashion and producing many errors.

MA Mental age.

masking effect The fact that one condition in a person may be strong enough to hide another entirely different condition which is present also. In children a low level of basic ability may mask dyslexic difficulties.

mental age (MA) An attempt to measure the amount of learning experiences a person has had in life. A calculation is made using both the person's chronological age (CA) and their intelligence level (IQ) in order to get as exact an age as possible.

mind blindness A term used by Morgan at the end of the 19th century to describe dyslexia.

mixed (dyseidetic/dysphonetic) dyslexia A sub-group of dyslexic children described by Boder. Children in this group show symptoms that are a mixture of the *dyseidetic* and the *dysphonetic* groups.

morphemic dyslexia Another term for the surface dyslexia, found in children, being one of two types described by Snowling. (The other sub-group is *phonological dyslexia*).

multi-sensory A method of teaching which employs as many of the senses as possible. When learning letters children can listen to its sound (HEARING), look at it in print (VISION), handle a plywood cut-out shape of it (TOUCH) and also trace the outline with a finger (KINAESTHETIC).

NAS/UWT National Association of School Masters/Union of Women Teachers.

National Curriculum In 1988 the Education Reform Act introduced a National Curriculum to be used in all county, voluntary, maintained special and grant-maintained schools. This was the first time any such action had been taken in the history of British Education. It began to be phased in over a number of years commencing in 1989. There are core subjects (Maths, English, Science) and foundation subjects (History, Geography, Technology, Art, Music, Physical Education and a Modern Foreign Language.) The National Curriculum is delivered over a 12-year period in four key stages:- (1) = 5–7 yrs, (2) = 8–11 yrs, (3) = 12–14 yrs and (4) = 15–16 yrs. The years are called, in order, R, 1, 2 and so on up to year 11. Assessments are carried out close to the end of each Key Stage and compared with the Attainment Targets expected to be achieved at that key stage. Reports are supplied to parents.

NCET National Council for Educational Technology.

nerve cell The basic unit or building block of the body's nervous system, the medical term for such a cell being NEURONE. They vary in size from as small as 3 micrometres to over 1 metre and have three parts (cell body, dendrites, axon). The basic purpose is to convey 'messages' from one part of the body to another. See also *nerve fibre*.

nerve fibre The axon of a nerve cell (neurone), together with its surrounding membrane, is known as a nerve fibre.

neurologist One who studies neurology, which is concerned with the structure and function of the nervous system.

neuropsychology The study of the interrelationship between behaviour and the nervous system.

NFER National Foundation for Educational Research.

normal curve The shape of a graph which results when the distribution of some property (or aspect) of a population is plotted. The shape is derived from probability theory with most scores being clustered about an average (mean) value and scores very different from the mean occurring far less often. Height and weight are examples of what yield a normal curve, as are speeds of running or swimming.

occipital lobe Each hemisphere of the brain has an occipital lobe which is the rearmost of the four.

optic chiasma Located in the brain and part of the visual pathway, it is the place where the two inside bundles of optic nerve fibres from the back of the eye cross-over. In front of the optic chiasma are the *optic nerves* and behind them are the *optic tracts*.

optic radiations Part of the visual pathway of the brain and located between the *lateral geniculate nucleus* and the *occipital lobes* each of the two optic radiations transmits visual information from the former to the latter. The nerves of the optic radiations form a distinct pattern.

optic tracts Part of the visual pathway of the brain and located immediately behind the *optic chiasma*. Each optic tract (there are two – one in each half of the brain) consists of nerves from the outside half of the eye on the same side of the brain as itself, together with those from the inside half of the other eye.

organic books Also called '*real books*', they are written in a different style from *inorganic books* (which are the ones that have traditionally been used to teach reading). The aim of organic books is to tell a story in a way which will attract children and encourage them to learn to read. They sound well when read aloud, the language being more natural and with a more natural 'flow' to it.

parietal lobe One of the four lobes which make up each half of the brain. Its location is above the temporal lobe and between the frontal and occipital lobes.

PATOSS Professional Association of Teachers of Students with Specific Learning Difficulties.

PEP Principal Educational Psychologist.

phoneme The smallest unit of sound which can distinguish one word from another, e.g. pan – ban, or cat – cot. Normal English makes use of 44 phonemes, 24 being consonants and 20 being vowels. When English is written down the fact that there are only 26 letters in the alphabet to represent 44 different sounds means that some letters, used singly or in pairs, need to represent more than one sound. This is a complication that children have to overcome in learning to read.

phonemic analysis The process of analysing the sound of a word into the smaller sounds (phonemes) which form it.

phonemic awareness The realisation that a word is not a single 'block' of sound but is made up of a collection of smaller sounds (phonemes). When learning to read a child must be able to analyse a word into its component sounds and then synthesise (or blend) them together to produce the spoken word. See *phonemic analysis, phonemic synthesis*.

phonemic segmentation Another name for *phonemic analysis*.

phonemic synthesis The process of building up a word from the smaller sounds (phonemes) from which it is composed.

phonetics The scientific study of the sounds involved in speech production generally (compare with *phonology*).

phonics (i) A method of teaching reading and spelling. It is based on the sounding-out of each letter (or grouping of letters) in a word. It is to be contrasted with the *look-and-say* method. (ii) An obsolete term for *phonetics* (used in the 17th century).

phonological dyslexia (i) A sub-grouping of the *acquired dyslexia* found in adults. It is described as being similar to *deep dyslexia* but less pronounced in intensity. A person who is a phonological dyslexic has difficulty with non-words and the sounding out of words generally. Visual errors are quite likely to occur but there is less chance of errors related to word meanings. (ii) A sub-grouping of the *developmental dyslexia* found in children. It was one of two types proposed by Snowling in 1987, the other being *surface (or morphemic) dyslexia*. Children who are phonological dyslexics are described as resembling phonologically dyslexic adults in their reading and spelling.

phonological processor dyslexia A sub-grouping of the developmental dyslexia found in children, one of three sub-groups proposed by Seymour (1986). He found evidence of phonological weakness in all his dyslexic subjects. The other two sub-groupings he proposed are *semantic processor* and *visual processor dyslexics*.

phonology The study of the speech sounds of a particular language (compare with *phonetics*).

pictogram (often referred to as pictograph) A symbol used in picture writing, e.g. a set of wavy lines might represent the sea or a river.

pilot study A study which is carried out before the main study is undertaken and which is intended as a trial run in order to identify any possible future difficulties etc. while there is still time to carry out improvements of design.

pre-reading skills Those skills considered beneficial to a child when about to be taught reading, e.g. the ability to listen to stories, to be able to distinguish between one sound and another, or one shape and another, to compare and contrast, to order and arrange, to draw and paint etc.

pro forma A document with blanks to be filled in.

PSP Parental Support Project.

'P'-type dyslexia One of two sub-groups of dyslexic children, the other being 'L' type as claimed by Bakker in 1990. He claims that 60–70% of dyslexic children fall into one or other of these sub-groups. A 'P' type of dyslexic child is described as reading relatively slower and in a fragmented fashion, albeit rather accurately as they remain sensitive to the perceptual features of text.

RA Reading age.

raw score A number which usually shows how many questions/ tasks/items a child got correct in a test. It is simply a quantity that has little if any meaning as it needs to be converted into a *scaled score*. This will give an indication of the quality of the test results obtained by comparing them with those from many other children of the same age.

'real' books Another name for *'organic books'*.

rebus A picture or symbol which represents a word or phrase. Many road signs consist of a rebus, e.g. a red and black car side by side within a red circle means 'no overtaking', a human figure holding a spade means 'road works ahead' etc. (A child with reading difficulties might respond to a scheme which employs rebuses).

received pronunciation (RP) Pronunciation that is regarded as correct or proper. RP should be understood by all who use the language and should also be the pronunciation taught to foreigners who are learning the language.

retarded Held back, made slow or late on arriving is the literal meaning. In the case of a child's reading progress the use of the word retarded implies that the child is capable of reading at a higher level but that some circumstances (e.g. deafness) are preventing him from doing so. There is also the implication that once the cause of the retardation is removed then the child will make progress at the expected rate. Retardation is measured by comparing what the child is expected to achieve (the mental age) with what he is actually achieving. It is to be contrasted with *backwardness*. (Confusion sometimes arises as in the USA retarded is used in the same sense that backward is used in Great Britain).

retina The light-sensitive layer at the back of the eye which is composed of the highly specialised *rod* and *cone* cells and on to which images of the outside world are focused by the *lens*.

rods One of the two specialised cells in the retina of the eye, the other being the *cones*. There are 120 million rods in each eye and they respond to differences in light and shade.

RP Received pronunciation.

SALVA See-And-Learn-Visual-Aid.

scaled score The meaningful score into which the *raw score* of a test is converted. It is meaningful as it produces a figure which can be compared with that produced by large numbers of other children of the same age and so can give an insight into whether a child has a particular difficulty and, if so, how serious it is likely to be.

semantic processor dyslexia A sub-grouping of the developmental dyslexia found in children, one of three sub-groups proposed by Seymour (1986). However he found that his data could not 'easily be put into a coherent scheme of sub-types'.

SEN Special educational needs.

SENCO Special Educational Needs Coordinator.

small (letter) Also known as '*lower case*' to distinguish from *capital* or '*upper case*'.

SNAP Special Needs Action Programme.

'soft' signs (of brain damage) Features such as coordination difficulties, abnormal reflex actions or an unusual EEG pattern. There could also be a mild degree of speech impairment or a difficulty with balance.

SOS Simultaneous Oral Spelling.

specific developmental dyslexia One of the many terms used to describe the form of dyslexia found in children. (It was defined by the World Federation of Neurology in 1968).

specific dyslexia A short form of *specific developmental dyslexia*.

specific learning difficulties (SpLD) The term which is preferred by many educational psychologists, teachers and researchers to describe *dyslexia* in children. (It was defined by Tansley and Panckhurst in 1981 and by the Dyslexia Institute in 1989).

specific reading difficulties One of the many terms used to describe *dyslexia* in children. It was used by the DES in 1972 in one of its reports which had resulted from the formation of the Advisory Committee for Handicapped Children (Chairman – Professor J. Tizard). The report was entitled *Children with Specific Reading Difficulties*).

specific reading disabilities One of the many terms used to describe *dyslexia* in children.

specific reading retardation One of the many terms used to describe *dyslexia* in children. (It was defined by Rutter, Tizard and Whitmore in 1970).

SPELD *Spe*cific *L*earning *D*ifficulties – which stands for a movement set up in New South Wales in 1967 and must *not* be confused with SpLD.

SpLD Specific learning difficulties. (This should not be confused with SLD which stands for severe learning difficulties.)

SPS Schools Psychological Service.

SS Social Services.

SSS Scotopic Sensitivity Syndrome.

standardise This refers to the process of transforming the rough (or raw) results of testing into units of measurement which are meaningful. The outcome is that the standardised scores can be compared in a meaningful way with scores from a different test, e.g. a score of 48 out of 100 on one test can be compared with 37 out of 60 on another even if one was marked more severely than another.

strephosymbolia Literally, 'the twisting of symbols'. An early term to describe dyslexia.

sulcus A shallow cleft on the brain's surface. Being of Latin origin, the plural form is sulci.

surface dyslexia (i). A sub-group of the acquired dyslexia found in adults. Surface dyslexics are able to read phonetically regular words and non-words. However, they have difficulties with irregular words and cannot make use of visual analysis to recognise whole words. The surface dyslexic over-relies on phonological methods, slowly sounding out the words as he reads. (ii) Also known as *morphemic dyslexia*, surface dyslexics are a sub-grouping of children described by Snowling in 1987. (The other sub-grouping is *phonological dyslexia*). The children who are surface dyslexics are described as being similar to adults with surface dyslexia.

SW Social worker.

syllabification The process of breaking down a word into its syllables.

syllable A part of a word, distinguishable from the other part(s) by the sounds of speech. Each syllable must have either one vowel, two or more vowels in combination, or the letter y in it. There may be consonants in addition but the foregoing is essential. There is one syllable in: *dog, soup, sky*, two syllables in:- *water, monkey, welcome*, and three syllables in: *happiness, wonderful, tidily*. Syllables are themselves made up of *phonemes*.

syntax The way in which words are arranged grammatically to show relationships and meaning within a sentence.

temporal lobe One of the four lobes of each cerebral hemisphere. It is at the side of the head, in the region of the temple (hence the name) and lies below the lateral fissure.

traumatic dyslexia Another name for *acquired dyslexia* in adults.

UKRA United Kingdom Reading Association.

upper-case (letters) A printer's term for *capital letters*, as opposed to *small* (or *lower-case*) *letters*.

ventricle A small cavity in the brain filled with cerebrospinal fluid. There are four in all.

visual dyslexia Claimed to be a sub-type of both *alexia* and *developmental dyslexia* and, together with auditory dyslexia, is one of the earliest sub-types to be identified. A visual dyslexic has difficulty in recognising the appearance of a word on the basis of how the word sounds. 'Auditory methods' of teaching are claimed to produce the best results. Many make comparisons between visual dyslexia, dyseidetic dyslexia and the visual-grapheme processor dyslexia.

visual pathway The route taken by nerve impulses as they travel from the rear of the eyes to the visual cortex at the back of the brain. The parts involved are, in order: the *retinas*, the *optic nerves*, the *optic chiasma*, the *optic tracts*, the *lateral geniculate nuclei*, the *optic radiations* and the *occipital lobes*.

visual processor dyslexia A sub-grouping of the developmental dyslexia found in children, one of three proposed by Seymour in 1986. (The other two sub-groups he proposed are *semantic processor* and *phonological processor* dyslexics. After carrying out his study he felt that the results could not 'easily be fitted into a coherent scheme of sub-types'.

vitreous humour The clear, jelly-like substance which fills most of the eyeball and which lies between the lens and the retina.

WAIS Wechsler Adult Intelligence Scale.

white matter The bulk of the material which goes to make up the brain. It lies beneath the 3 mm thick '*grey matter*' or *cerebral cortex* but in the spine is on the outside of the grey matter. It is mainly composed of nerve fibres.

Whole-Word (Method of Teaching Reading) Another name for the *look-and-say* method.

WISC Wechsler Intelligence Scale for Children.

word blindness One of the first names given to dyslexia and, despite the passage of more than a century, one which is still quite popular in the public mind.

WPPSI Wechsler Pre-School and Primary Scale of Intelligence.

Index